1 Fit Self-Improvement Series
FIGURE MAINTENANCE

1 Fit Self-Improvement Series
FIGURE MAINTENANCE

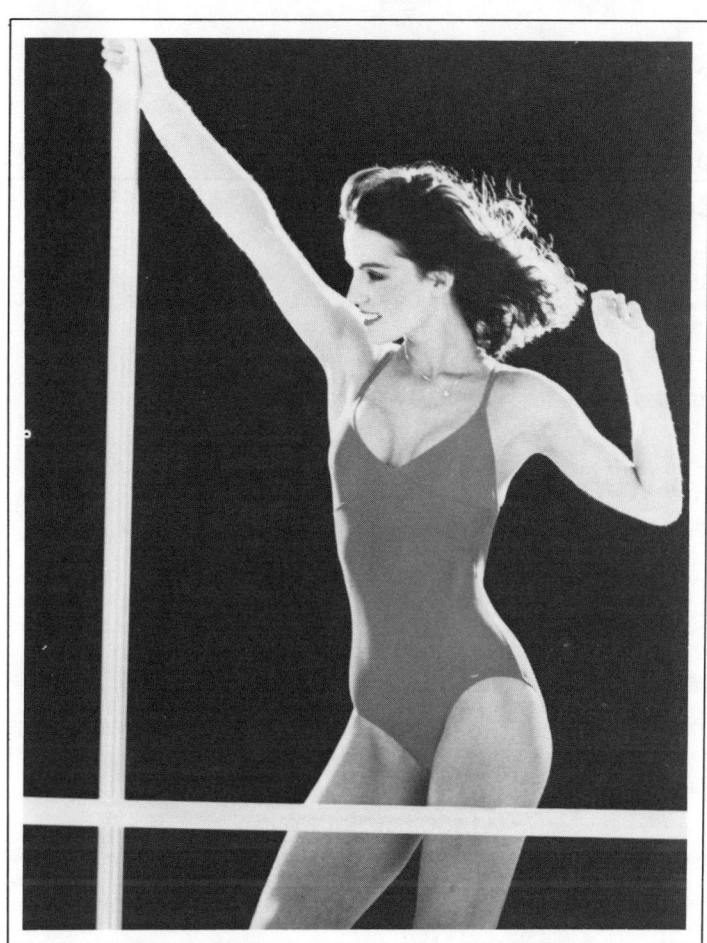

by Catherine Cassidy
and the editors of *FiT*

ANDERSON WORLD BOOKS, INC.

Library of Congress Cataloging in Publication Data
Cassidy, Catherine, 1959—
  Figure maintenance.
  (Fit self-improvement series; 1)
  1. Women — Health and hygiene.   2. Physical fitness for women. 3. Beauty, Personal.
I. Fit magazine. II. Title. III. Series.
RA778.C227   1983   613'.04244   83-2734
ISBN 0-89037-255-1

No information in this book may be reproduced in any form
without permission from the publisher.
Anderson World, Inc.
1400 Stierlin Road
Mountain View, CA
94043
©1983, by
Anderson World, Inc.

CONTENTS

INTRODUCTION	vii
1 DIET	1
2 EXERCISE	27
3 STAYING HEALTHY	51
4 STRESS AND RELAXATION	55
5 APPEARANCE	65
BIBLIOGRAPHY	83
CREDITS	85

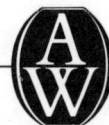

INTRODUCTION

A Letter to Myself

"Wait a minute. Have I thought about fitness today? I like to consider myself a fit person. I watch what I eat. I exercise regularly (I think). And I feel good about myself.

"Or am I just telling myself that to make me feel better? To justify that luscious dessert I had last night? Am I passing up the chance to go out for a quick, refreshing run by looking in the mirror and telling myself, 'Oh, you look okay; you don't need to run today . . . ?'

"If I want to look good and feel good all the time, I have to think about looking good and feeling good all the time. I have to remember that fitness, health, and beauty, are not conditions that I can achieve by simply dieting for a month, or by playing volleyball at lunch once a week. And I can't put on makeup to feign health. If I want to be a really fit person, then I have to act like a really fit person. I have to always watch what I eat; I have to exercise, at least four days a week. If I don't, then I am selling myself short.

"Fitness is an ongoing process . . . it's a commitment, a lifelong commitment. And if I want to be fit, I have to realize that. I have to make goals for myself, every day, and do my best to achieve them.

"It's hard work, but do I really want to be a fit, attractive woman?"

Right now, grab a piece of paper and a pencil and write that little letter out in your own handwriting. Don't scribble it; write it neatly, so that you can read it very quickly. Then tack it up on the door of your refrigerator, so that you can see it every time you walk into the kitchen.

Sound like nonsense? It's not. Being fit truly is hard work. It takes discipline to have a lifestyle that includes fitness. That's because fitness isn't a characteristic you're born with, and it's not something that you can buy through a mail-order catalog or through a fad diet. Fitness is a lifestyle. It involves a lot of behavior modification, or changing your habits to include practices that are healthy — like getting out of bed at 6 a.m. instead of 6:45 so that you can take a quick three-mile run or do a few aerobic exercises in the living room. Or like passing up the McDonald's restaurant after a Saturday-morning shopping spree and instead making a tuna fish sandwich at home.

Fitness involves making a lot of sacrifices, too. That homemade tuna sandwich may not be quite as tempting as a juicy hamburger and a chocolate shake, and it takes a little bit of self-prodding to drive past that McDonald's without a second thought. And you may not want to rise at the crack of dawn with the birds when you could get almost an hour more of shut-eye, but if that's the only time you can exercise, then that's the sacrifice you'll have to make — if you want to be fit.

It's easy to thumb through a lot of health and fitness magazines, gaze enviously at the gorgeous, shapely models in the photos and say with a sigh, "Well, *I* certainly couldn't ever be like them. Why don't those magazines use models that look more like real people?" Surprise! They are real people, and do you know how they got to be so beautiful? Not by sitting around on their fannies all day and gorging themselves on fattening foods. Those models watch their weight very carefully, every single day. They exercise their tails off every day, too, because they know that if they don't, they'll lose that shapely figure and that glowing complexion that the camera captures so vividly. They work at fitness and beauty almost every day of the year.

There — the secret's out. But fitness really isn't a secret — it's just difficult work, which is why most women in America today are not fit. The tide is turning, however, and the '80s have ushered in a new awareness of health and fitness that has really started to get people going — people like yourself, who are ready to tackle the responsibility of keeping themselves fit and healthy.

A lot of women do have the gumption to get on the track toward fitness, but don't know how to get started with their programs. That's a common problem, and many times women get discouraged because they don't have the money to join an expensive health spa or exercise program, which is a popular way. Half the time, that discouragement will set them back far enough as to make them abandon their goals altogether.

Well, that's just not a good enough reason to stay dumpy and out of shape. You really don't need a lot of money to be fit, just a lot of determination, a little bit of common sense, and a knowledge of what it takes to be fit, and to maintain that fitness.

Your Body Is Like Your Car

"Now what's that supposd to mean?" you are probably asking yourself. "What does my car have to do with my body?"

Well, literally speaking, next to nothing — most of us do not look like cars (although at times we may feel as though we've been hit by a Mack truck), and most of us don't wish to look like cars. But many women know as much about their bodies as they do about their cars — next to nothing.

When we received our driver's licenses at the tender age of sixteen (or whenever), we hopped right in behind the wheel and drove off into the sunset. Unfortunately, most of us did not know the first thing about the machine we were licensed to drive. If you've ever been to the auto mechanic, this ignorance probably hindered you. "Yes," we would say, "There was this knocking somewere, and all of a sudden my car wouldn't start." The mechanic would smile wryly and say, "We'll take care of it, lady," and the next thing you knew, you were paying the bill, usually a big bill. You had no idea what he did; perhaps you still didn't even know what was wrong with your car. You didn't realize that if you don't put water in the battery, it will die, or if you don't get a tune-up every once in a while, your car will stall at every stoplight. You never found out about any of this until it was too late.

Many women are as uneducated about their bodies as they are about their cars. They never find out what's going on inside until it's too late. They've gotten fat and soft because of overeating the wrong foods, out of shape because they don't exercise, sick because they smoke and drink too much. And like their cars, they pay a pretty price.

But unlike cars, that body can't be replaced if it's been neglected too long. However wretched-looking and sickly it may be, that body is yours for life. So it really makes sense to take care of it once in a while.

There's also a difference between being "drivable" and being "in great shape." You can drive an old car with an ailing muffler and a weary engine: It just won't get you as far, as fast. As any high-school-age jalopy owner can tell you, you have to service it all the time in order to keep that car of yours in prime condition.

The same is true of your body. You could live on a diet of burgers and shakes if you were so inclined; many do. And you could get by even if the only exercise you did was opening and closing the refrigerator door. The body is an incredibly adaptable machine. It can take loads of abuse and still manage to perform — up to a point. It won't look half as nice as it could if you took good care of it conscientiously, and it won't last as long.

Think about it. If you wanted to, you really could compare your body to your car. Look at your diet. Isn't the food you eat something like the fuel you put into your car? If you use cheap fuel, your car is going to knock; it sounds like there's a woodpecker making a nest under your hood. Without high-quality fuel, your car is just not going to perform as well as it might.

And that oil in your car — you can compare that to your diet, too. You've got to use a high-grade oil to keep that auto of yours in top working condition, and if you don't have it changed regularly, if you let it get too dirty, it will gum up the works. If you let your diet get too "dirty," too full of fatty foods and empty sugar and starch calories, you're going to gum up the works of your body. And you could end up overweight, at best, or at worst, with heart disease.

And that word *maintenance:* It's important to your car, and it's important to your body, too. So you use the highest grade oil, and you've got steel-belted radials, a good suspension system, good brakes and a good reliable engine. How long is everything going to be "good" unless you maintain it? Not very long. Those brakes are going to get spongy and start to squeal, those tires are going to wear down, and that engine is going to give you problems. Maintaining a car is a regular job, whether you do it yourself or have an auto mechanic do it for you.

The same goes for your body, as you might have guessed. That good diet of yours won't be worth a hoot unless you assist your body in making the most of all the good foods you eat. Body maintenance means knowing how it works and making sure it works — through exercise. Thirty minutes of exercise four to six days a week is the best possible maintenance your body could ask for, and it will thank you for your time by being strong, healthy and in tip-top shape.

But all of this is easy to generalize about. And it's easy to write "I will make a commitment to fitness" and tack it up on the refrigerator door. It's a little more difficult to actually *make* that commitment, unless you know how to go about doing it. But if you think you've got the guts to try for a fit lifestyle, the next few chapters of this book show you how to achieve and maintain a fit, healthy figure.

1 DIET

THE PROPER FUEL: THE IMPORTANCE OF A GOOD DIET

Yes, again. No matter how many times you've heard it all before, diet is just about the most important factor to consider when it comes to staying fit and healthy. And it indeed warrants being brought up one more time. That old saying "You are what you eat" couldn't be more accurate — or more discouraging, if your diet is filled with junk food.

But what is "junk food"? People are really confused these days about what to eat and what not to eat. It's easy to choose fuel for your car — it's got to be one of three: leaded, unleaded (regular or premium) or diesel. But food is a little bit different. You can't just walk into Safeway and ask for an unleaded diet. You have to choose the food you eat, and, for what it's worth, you have millions of choices.

It's not always easy to make the right choices, either. Even nutrition experts don't agree on what the perfect, balanced diet should consist of, so it's almost impossible for the consumer to know.

But by making your commitment to a fit, healthy lifestyle, you have also agreed (whether you know it or not) to go in search of a better diet for yourself. The number of people who need to do so is staggering. According to the American Dietetic Association, more than eighty million Americans, both men and women, are considered overweight by their doctors. That's about 36 percent of our population! And that's probably not even taking into consideration all those men and women sitting at home who haven't been to the doctor recently. The reason that most of those people are overweight in the first place is poor diet — inadequate nutrition, as the experts call it.

But let's say you're not overweight. Should you still watch your diet? You'd better, because a poor diet manifests itself in more ways than just excess fat. What your diet really affects is inside of you. Those burgers and that chocolate shake are broken down in your small intestines into chemicals that can be easily absorbed into the bloodstream. From there, those chemicals travel to every part of your body, nourishing the cells and tissue.

So it is wise to feed all those cells properly. If your diet doesn't contain enough of the essential nutrients the cells need to build and repair themselves, you will wind up built like a house of cards. Your body will be more vulnerable to stress and more susceptible to disease.

Diet affects how you feel, too. A poor diet can make you nervous and irritable, or leave you feeling tired and run down and just not feeling up to par. And even though you might not be overweight, diet can really damage your appearance. A lot of those hungry cells live on

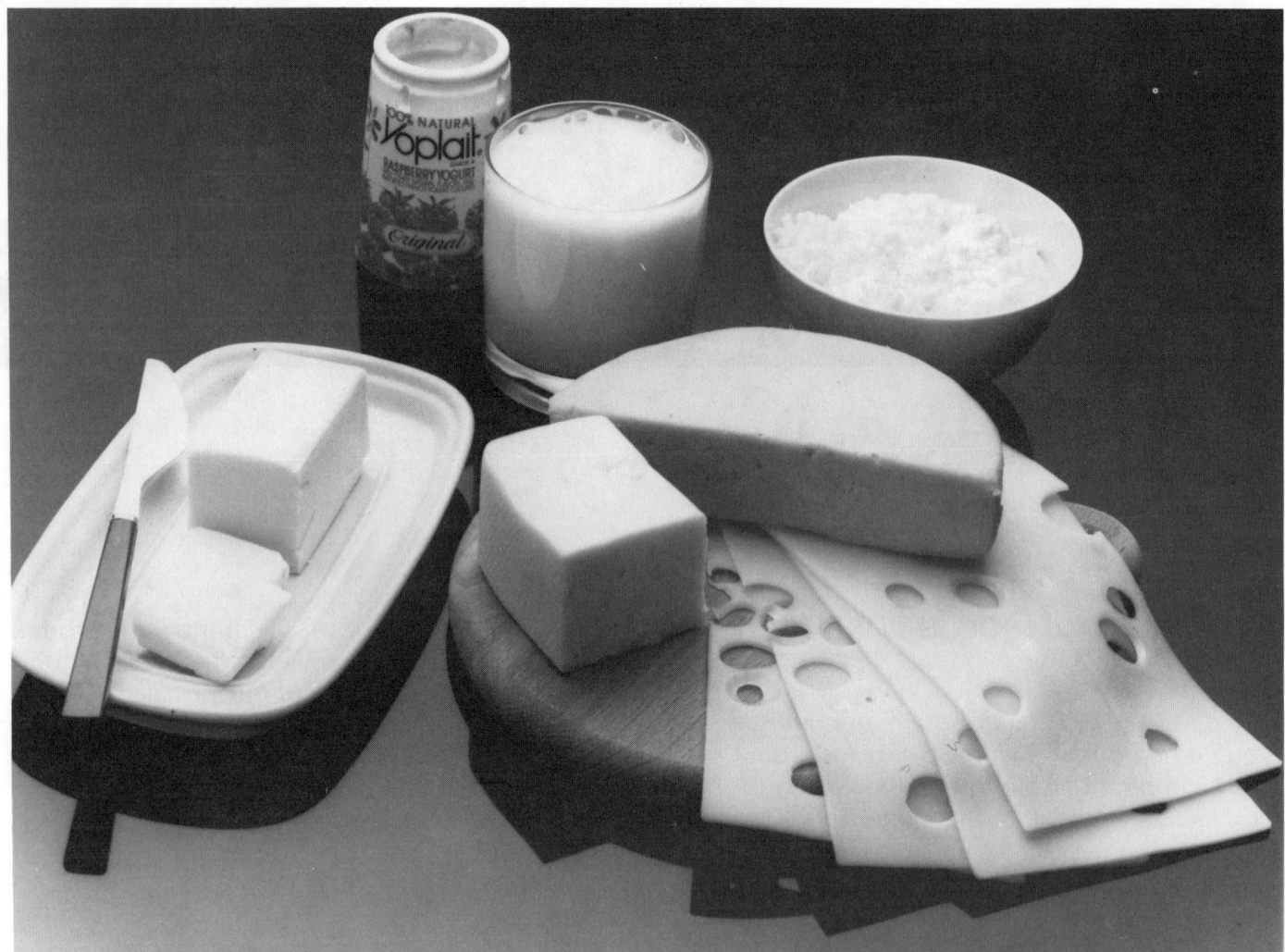

The Dairy Group includes milk and butter.

the surface of your body, and the condition of your hair, skin and fingernails is a good indication of how well you're eating. Hair that is dull and lifeless, fingernails that are brittle and splitting, and skin that is dry or colorless are all common signs of some nutritional deficiency.

And though you may not be overweight, look in the mirror. How is your posture? Posture can also be adversely affected by a poor diet, which affects the strength of the muscles and bones; if your muscles aren't strong enough to support the weight of the rest of your body, they can lead to poor posture. One of the most common problems of old age is a condition called osteoporosis, wherein the bones have lost considerable calcium. This leaves them porous and brittle, and more susceptible to fractures. There is considerable evidence suggesting that some cases of osteoporosis are caused directly by a lack of calcium and other essential nutrients in the diet.

So it is important to watch your diet. But don't be scared into eating foods that are good for you; know that a proper, healthy diet is a positive thing. When you eat right, you look good, and you feel good, too. And that's what being fit is all about.

So where should you start in your search for better nutrition? Actually, although supermarkets are laden with a gaggle of nutritionless foods, you can still find the proper fuel for your body, provided you know what "proper fuel" is.

THE BASIC FOUR

We all heard, as small children, about the importance of the four food groups. Well, times have changed little as far as nutrition is concerned, and those same basic four are still the building blocks of a good diet. It is how you put those basic four together that makes all the

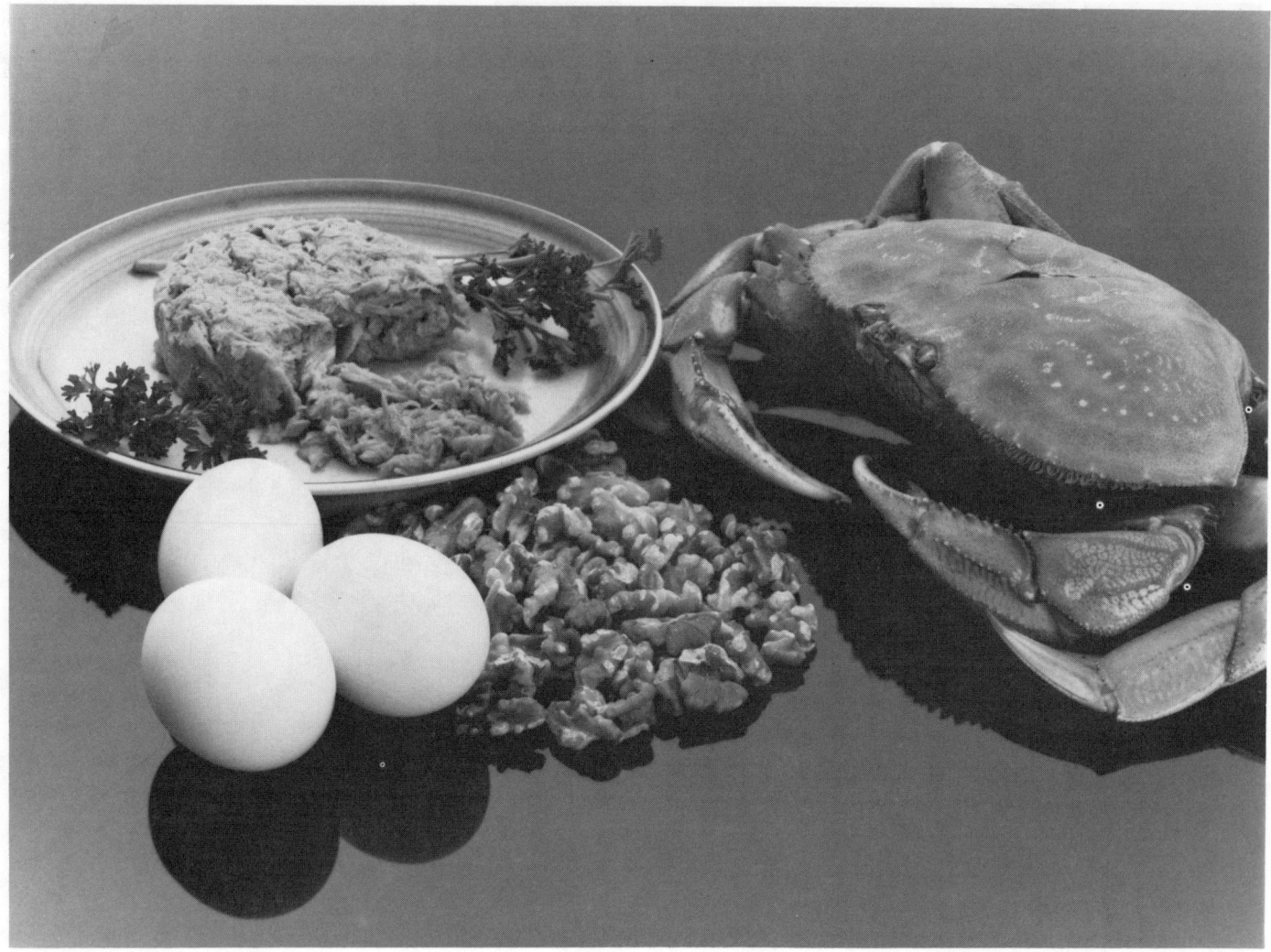

High-protein foods make up the Meat Group.

difference. One of the keys to good nutrition is variety, and the other is balance. It's not really practical, or even possible, to sit down with complicated nutrition charts and plan out every meal that will follow precise nutritional guidelines. But you can, by putting together meals from these four food groups, assure yourself of a fairly well-balanced and nutritious diet.

Dairy Products

There is much controversy today surrounding this group of foods, particularly milk itself. People have been led to believe that foods from this group should be avoided, because they are high in fat. It is true; a person can drink too much milk, if that person is replacing other necessary foods with milk. But don't overcompensate by avoiding milk products completely (unless you are instructed to do so by a doctor or nutrition specialist). While milk is high in fat, it also is an important source of high-quality protein, calcium, phosphorus and vitamin D, all of which are necessary for a well-balanced diet.

If you are worried about the fat content of whole milk, switch to low-fat or skim milk instead. Yogurt, cottage cheese and buttermilk are other good sources of these essential nutrients that are fairly low in calories. A good diet should include some foods from this group.

Meats

Meats are an important source of complete protein and they also provide an abundant supply of essential vitamins and minerals. Most people rely on this food group for the protein in their diets; however, as vegetarians will attest, meats are not the only source of protein. Dairy products, as mentioned before, are also high in protein, and a combination of whole grains and legumes (which we will discuss later) can provide complete protein.

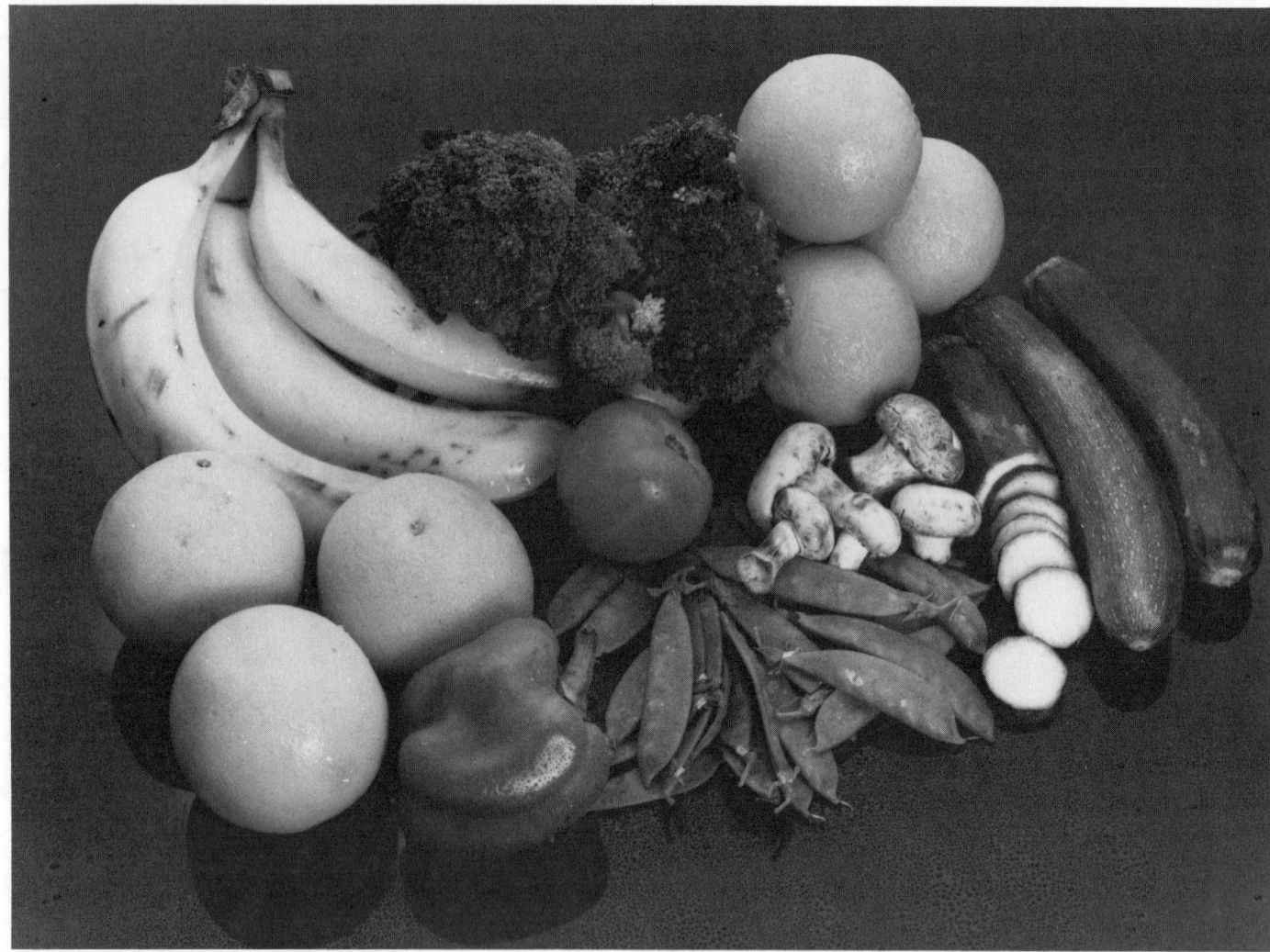
Fruits and vegetables are high in vitamin C.

If you are a meat eater, though, include lean meats in your diet, meats like chicken, other poultry, fish, eggs (although they are not a meat, they are complete proteins like meat) and very lean beef products. Many people steer clear of red meat, and for good reason. Red meat is not as easily digested by your system because of its high fat content. If you are a red-meat eater, make sure the cuts you choose are the leanest possible.

And for heaven's sake, stay away from those preserved meats like bologna, wieners and other lunchmeats. They are full of just that — preservatives — and your body does not need preservatives.

Fruits and Vegetables

These are wonderful foods! And, unfortunately, many people just don't realize what a storehouse of nutrients they are. We were always told when we were young to eat all of our vegetables, and for some reason, it was a deplorable task. We found it much easier to feed our vegetables to the family dog than to eat them ourselves.

For some reason, this thinking seems to have followed us from our youth into adulthood. When it comes to vegetables, we are always looking for ways to hide them: burying them in butter and salt, buying them canned or frozen and mixing them into casseroles, or choking them in heavy creams and sauces.

Sadly, all of this cooking and fussing hides the great natural taste of vegetables, and saps them of most of their nutrients as well. Vegetables (and fruits) have little, if any, fat, and are veritable storehouses of an assortment of vitamins and minerals. But boiling, baking and generally overcooking them will render them just about worthless, nutritionally speaking.

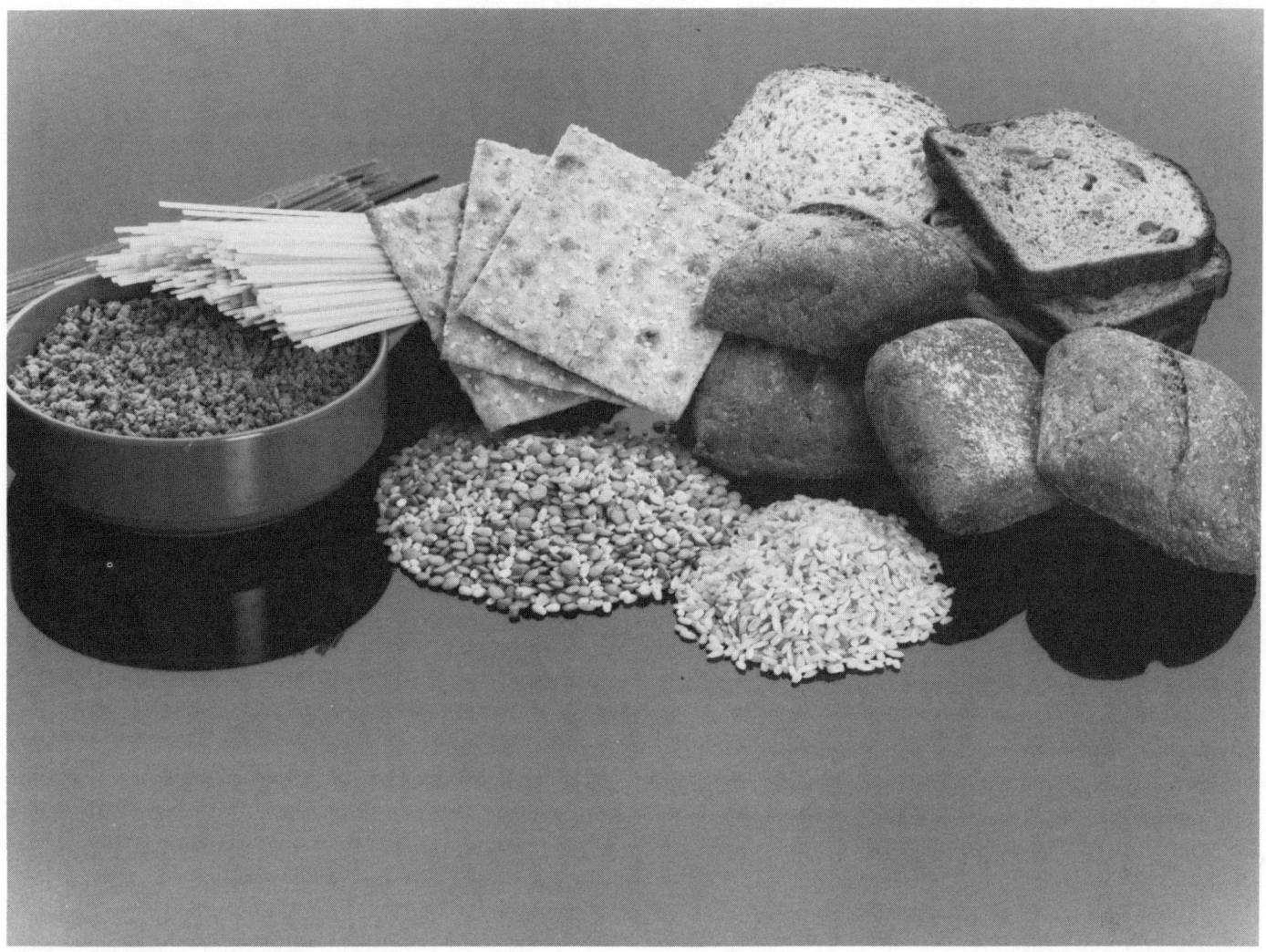
Grains are a source of many B vitamins.

Don't be afraid of vegetables! Include plenty of them in your diet. . . And don't overcook. Just steam them briefly; this preserves their vitamins and minerals and allows you to enjoy their fresh, natural taste.

And be a salad eater. Raw vegetables, besides supplying all those vitamins and minerals, are rich in natural enzymes and fiber, both of which are essential to proper digestion. And besides, they taste great.

Some of the vegetables you might choose from are green, leafy vegetables, roots (like turnips, carrots, beets, onions and yams), potatoes, gourds (squashes) and legumes (peas and beans).

Fruits are more widely accepted fare, but we still have found the need to load them up with sugar and put them in cans. As with vegetables, go fresh! Fresh fruits are excellent sources of all sorts of nutrients, ranging from vitamin C to potassium. Don't overload on them, though. Fruits contain sugar, in the form of natural fructose, and if you eat too many bananas, the result will manifest itself on your hips and thighs.

Whole Grains

There was a common belief in our family a few years back that whole wheat bread was unsuitable for eating; only little old ladies with constipation ate whole wheat bread. Kind of sad, but for many years, this was the feeling all across the country. Along with the refined milling processes developed early in this century came the feeling that anything except clean, white bread was "dirty" and wouldn't taste good.

This, of course, is nonsense. Actually, the parts that are generally discarded in the milling process, the germ and the bran, are two of the most important components of the grain, from a nutritional standpoint. The germ is probably the most nutritious portion of the grain, containing B vitamins, protein, unsaturated fat, minerals and carbohydrates. And the bran is an important source of fiber and trace elements. The part that you're left eating is generally devoid of nutrients, unless those nutrients have been replaced artificially.

The biggest fallacy of all, though, is the idea that whole grains don't taste good. They're delicious! And even though there is a proliferation of refined flour and grain products on the supermarket shelves, you can still find whole grains. Whole grain and whole seed breads, whole grain cereals and flours, and unhulled grains like brown rice, barley and millet are all delicious and nutritionally sound.

THE CASE FOR AND AGAINST FATS

Americans eat too much fat. According to recent government statistics, we consume 310 more calories of fat each day today than we did in the early part of this century. And we're fatter for it.

But all fats should not be eliminated from our diet. The body does need a certain amount of fat to maintain energy and to help the body transport the fat-soluble vitamins, like A, E, D and K, to different parts of the body. It just doesn't need as much as we feed it.

Average Fat Content of Typical Foods*

1.	Oils, shortenings	100%
2.	Butter, margarine	80%
3.	Most nuts	60%
4.	Peanut butter, bacon, donuts	50%
5.	Cheese, beef roasts	33%
6.	Lunch meat, franks	27%
7.	Lean pork, ice cream, cakes, pies	13%
8.	Most fish, lean lamb	7%
9.	Milk, shellfish, plain rolls	3%
10.	Most breads	1%

Shown as a percentage of total weight

Many people have been scared by the statistics involved with fats. And there are a lot of scary statistics. Overconsumption of saturated fat can help contribute to atherosclerosis, or hardening of the arteries, which in turn can lead to heart disease and stroke. And heart disease is one of the number one killers of Americans aged twenty-five and older. These facts have people running scared, and retaliating by removing all fats from their diets.

This is taking it too far. The key to maintaining a proper fat consumption is moderation, because taken in moderation, fats can promote health and, yes, beauty. Fats contribute sheen to the hair, silkiness and softness to the skin, and softness to bodily contours.

Unsaturated fats are usually liquid at room temperature and are derived from vegetables, seeds and nuts. Be sure your diet includes unsaturated fat, but not too much. The Recommended Daily Allowance of unsaturated fat is about two tablespoons. Saturated fats are the fats that have a lot of dieters in a whirl, but unless it has been recommended by your doctor, don't avoid products like milk, cheese and meats just because they contain fat. Use skim milk and trim the fat off your meat, but don't eliminate these foods entirely.

THOSE WONDERFUL VITAMINS

Vitamins have a somewhat strange yet very interesting history.

• During World War I, when men were out at sea for long periods of time, they developed what seemed to be acute rheumatism and tender, bleeding gums. The unknown disease was horrible; before the afflicted would die, they would swell up like balloons and suffer great pain. As soon as they were brought to shore and fed fresh fruit and vegetables, however, they were cured of these awful symptoms. "It's the vitamins!" nutritionists cried.

• In one Berlin hospital, children were dying of a dreadful disease called rickets, which softens the bones of infants, causing them to twist and become malformed, and can kill if left untreated. A doctor began to treat the children by tanning their skins with ultraviolet light — artificial sunshine. They were cured. "It's vitamin D! Vitamins cured them!" nutritionists exclaimed.

• In Japan, officers checked the spread of beriberi, a terrible, excruciatingly painful nerve disease, by feeding the sailors brown, unhulled rice instead of white rice. Beriberi was almost nonexistent on these ships. "It's the vitamins in the rice! The vitamins!" they all asserted.

• And in Africa, a British government official used lemon juice to cure natives dying of scurvy. "It's a vitamin!" was the response.

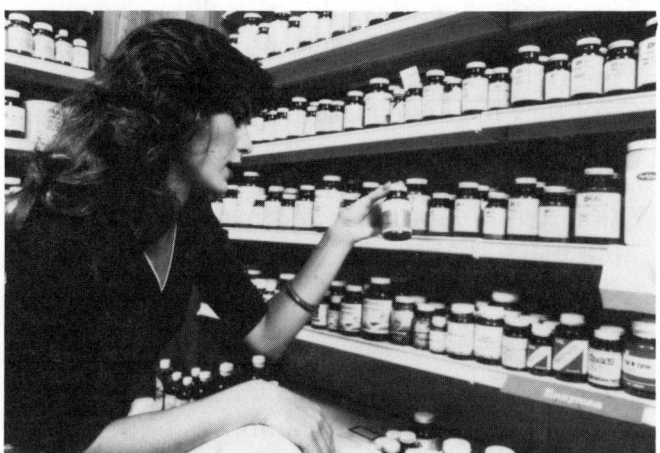

Study the label to determine the vitamins' potency.

Since the time when they received their first words of acclaim in the early part of this century, vitamins have been hailed as cure-alls and, more recently, life-prolongators. Vitamins are wonderful, indeed, and a certain amount of each vitamin and mineral is essential to your body. In fact, the lack of enough of these vitamins and minerals can cause illness, diseases, even death.

As was discovered in each of the previous examples, a small amount of a certain vitamin or mineral was enough to cure a disease that at one time would have wiped out an entire population. People soon went crazy with vitamins. And with this craze came a deluge of pills, pellets and powders, mineral supplements and combinations of every kind. No house was complete without its store of bottles of C, D, E and A. With the modern age of drugs, even the huge pharmaceutical companies couldn't resist getting in on the vitamin and mineral binge, and they came up with their own concoctions.

An entire generation was led to believe that its diet problems could be settled once and for all by taking the right doses of these wonderful vitamins.

Many people today are under that same impression — that enough vitamin pills will solve all of their diet problems. This is untrue. While vitamins represent an essential part of our diet, vitamin supplements cannot replace all the other essential nutrients that our diets may lack. Vitamins will not make up for a lack of good protein, or of fiber, for example. Vitamins are merely one element of a good, balanced diet.

And more often than not, we can get most of the vitamins we need from that good, balanced diet of ours, if foods are cooked properly and we make certain that we are eating the right kinds of foods. There are those who still endorse daily vitamin supplements: Jack La Lanne, for instance, takes more than four hundred himself, and Dr. Linus Pauling, whose research on vitamin C has earned him worldwide acclaim, believes in megadoses of C for everyone of every age.

So what should you do? First of all, get to know your diet intimately. What is the vitamin content of that carrot you're eating? Or that slice of bread? If you make an effort to meet all of your body's vitamin and mineral needs, chances are you won't have to supplement your diet drastically.

"But where do I get all those vitamins and minerals? I'm not sure if I'm eating the right foods. How can I tell?" Glad you asked. Here's a quick rundown of some of the vitamins and minerals you need, and how you can make sure your diet contains them:

Vitamin A — Vitamin A helps the body resist infection. Some deficiency signs include loss of appetite, dry hair, sudden onset of allergies, rough, dry skin, sinus problems and red, burning eyes. You can find this vitamin in green and yellow vegetables, milk, fish, carrots, apricots, eggs, lettuce, peaches and prunes.

Because B-complex vitamins are water-soluble (unlike vitamins A and E, which are fat

U.S. RECOMMENDED DAILY ALLOWANCES (R.D.A.s)

Vitamins, Minerals and Protein	Unit of Measurement	Adults	Pregnant or Lactating Women
*Vitamin A	International Units	5000	8000
Vitamin D	International Units	400	400
Vitamin E	International Units	30	30
*Vitamin C	Milligrams	60	60
Folic Acid	Milligrams	0.4	0.8
*Thiamine	Milligrams	1.5	1.7
*Riboflavin	Milligrams	1.7	2.0
*Niacin	Milligrams	20	20
Vitamin B-6	Milligrams	2.0	2.5
Vitamin B-12	Micrograms	6.0	8.0
Biotin	Milligrams	0.3	0.3
Pantothenic Acid	Milligrams	10	10
*Calcium	Grams	1.0	1.3
Phosphorus	Grams	1.0	1.3
Iodine	Micrograms	150	150
*Iron	Micrograms	18	18
Magnesium	Micrograms	400	450
Copper	Micrograms	2.0	2.0
Zinc	Micrograms	15	15

*Values of these nutrients must be declared on package labels. Listing of other vitamins and minerals is optional.
Source: Food and Drug Administration

Source: Runner's World Vitamin Book by Virginia De Moss (Anderson World Publications, 1982)

soluble), they are forever being washed out of our systems. Therefore, we have to take care that we replenish these important nutrients. Here are some of those most important B vitamins:

B₁ (Thiamine) — This has the shortest life of all the B vitamins in our body. It is also heat-sensitive, so cooking can damage it. B₁ helps us out by breaking down carbohydrates so that they can be used as energy. It also helps keep muscles more elastic, especially those in the circulatory and digestive systems. You can get your B₁ from wheat germ, brown rice, peanuts and brewer's yeast (most of the B vitamins can be obtained from brewer's yeast).

B₂ (Riboflavin) — Some food sources of this digestive aid are whole grains, beets, carrots, cottage cheese, milk, fish, green leafy vegetables and legumes (like beans or peas).

B₃ (Niacin) — Like other B vitamins, niacin promotes tissue health, especially in the liver, kidneys, heart, brain and muscles. Niacin also helps in the body's elimination of toxins and wastes. It can be found in milk, seafood, brown rice, peanuts, rhubarb and poultry, to name a few.

B₆ (Pyridoxine) — This vitamin is known for its importance in red blood cell production, but it also helps regulate hormone balance in the body. Women who are taking birth control pills may need extra B₆ to help them regulate their body chemistry, which can be interrupted by the pill. It helps control depression and nervousness and maintains sodium-potassium balance in the body. Some food sources are brown rice, whole grains, green leafy vegetables, legumes and liver.

B₁₂ (Colabamin) — This vitamin is crucial in red blood cell formation, and its presence also helps prevent anemia. B₁₂ has also been shown to provide extra resistance against germs and infection. Some sources of B₁₂ are whole grains, legumes, fish, milk, cheeses, chicken and eggs.

B₁₃ (Biotin) — Biotin is known as the "beauty vitamin" because of its marvelous effects on skin and hair. B₁₃ can be found in whole grains, legumes, eggs, sardines, brown rice.

Vitamin C (Ascorbic Acid) — Since vitamin C is water soluble and can't be stored, it must be replenished daily in the diet. The benefits of vitamin C are endless; to list them all would take at least two or three pages. Suffice it to say that without it, you most certainly would not be a healthy person. Vitamin C can be found in abundance in almost any fresh fruit or vegetable, with citrus fruits and — surprisingly — green peppers leading the pack.

Vitamin D — This vitamin is renowned for its role in maintaining healthy bones, teeth, nerves, skin and heart. Vitamin D is in eggs, bone meal, milk, salmon, tuna fish, citrus fruits, and other fruits and vegetables.

Vitamin E (Alpha-tocopherol) — Vitamin E can help increase the blood's oxygen-carrying capacity and guards against the wear and tear of stress. Vitamin E also plays an important role in preventing scarring and promoting healing. Vitamin E can be found in eggs, green leafy vegetables, corn, wheat germ, vegetable oils, safflower oil and peanuts.

Vitamin K (Menadione) — This element is essential to blood coagulation; without enough of it, you could bleed to death. To ensure that your diet includes enough vitamin K, include yogurt, safflower oil, green leafy vegetables, alfalfa sprouts, oatmeal or chicken livers in your diet.

THE MINERALS

Phosphorus — Phosphorus probably has more functions in the body than any other mineral. It is a major element in every body cell, and is essential in controlling the activity of the body's hormones, vitamins and enzymes. It is also necessary for digesting proteins, fats and carbohydrates, as well as a host of other bodily functions. Phosphorus can be found in legumes, eggs, nuts, fish, whole grains, poultry and yellow cheese.

Calcium — Calcium, too, is present in every body cell. It is essential for healthy bones and teeth, as most of us found out when we were very little, but it also plays a major role in cell division, muscle growth and contraction, and heart rhythm, among a host of other duties. Calcium can be found in alfalfa sprouts, blackstrap molasses, milk, cheese, yogurt and other milk products.

Copper — Yes, copper is an essential mineral to the body, not just a metal to make pennies out of. Copper's major function is as a catalyst in the body's healing process. Copper can be found in legumes, nuts, seafoods, soybeans, avocados and blackstrap molasses.

Iodine — Iodine is essential to metabolic regulation and thyroid hormone production. Iodine, as most people know, is available in iodized salt, but if you've chosen to eliminate salt from your diet, don't fret. You can get your iodine from seafood, kelp and mushrooms, too.

Potassium — Potassium is a key element in controlling the body's delicate equilibrium. It helps keep the brain supplied with oxygen and the kidneys functioning properly by acting as a diuretic to help flush toxic wastes from the body. It is also important to the health of the muscles. Potassium can be found in peaches, figs, dates, bananas, peanuts, potatoes, sunflower seeds, seafood and tomato juice.

Sodium — Sodium is essential to human nutrition, but can easily reach excess proportions in the body because of salt overuse or consumption of lots of processed foods, which are high in sodium. The best way to make sure you get enough sodium without getting too much is to lay off the salt shaker and the packaged and processed foods, and stick to the natural sources of this mineral like milk, cheeses, seafood and celery.

Iron — Iron is the prime carrier of oxygen in the bloodstream, and because women lose a good deal of blood each month through menstruation, they should pay particular attention to getting enough iron in their diets. Include plenty of green leafy vegetables, eggs, fish, poultry or blackstrap molasses in your diet to be certain that your body is getting its proper share of iron.

Magnesium — Magnesium helps strengthen bones and muscles, regulate body temperature and synthesize protein and vitamins. Magnesium can be found in bran, honey, green leafy vegetables, kelp, tuna fish and nuts.

Zinc — Zinc is important for building up protein stores, which make up most of the solid matter of the body's cells. Zinc is also required for normal growth and functioning of the liver, bones, skin, eyes, blood and nails. Zinc can be found in milk, whole grains, brown rice, legumes, poultry, nuts, fruits, cabbage, carrots and wheat germ.

ARE YOU COMING UP SHORT?

GROUP — **MAY HAVE LOWERED LEVELS OF:**

Group	A	Thiamin	Rib.	Niacin	B6	Folacin	B12
Elderly Women		•	•	•	•	•	•
Pregnant Women*	•	•			•	•	•
Nursing Women*		•				•	
Menstruating Women**							
Heavy Drinkers				•	•	•	
Users of Oral Contraceptives		•	•		•		•
Prolonged Users of Antibiotics		•					
Regular Users of Other Prescription Drugs	•				•		
Chronically Ill						•	
Heavy Smokers							
Persons with Disorders That Interfere with Fat Absorption***	•						
Gastrectomy Patients							
Post-operative and Burn Patients							
Vegans							
Fad Dieters and Persons on Strict Low-Calorie Diets****							

Group	Biotin	Pan. Acid	C	D	E	K	Calcium	Iron
Elderly Women		•	•	•			•	
Pregnant Women*			•					•
Nursing Women*								•
Menstruating Women**								•
Heavy Drinkers			•					
Users of Oral Contraceptives			•					
Prolonged Users of Antibiotics	•	•				•		
Regular Users of Other Prescription Drugs			•	•	•	•		
Chronically Ill			•					
Heavy Smokers			•					
Persons with Disorders That Interfere with Fat Absorption***				•	•	•		
Gastrectomy Patients								
Post-operative and Burn Patients			•					
Vegans								•
Fad Dieters and Persons on Strict Low-Calorie Diets****			•					•

*Doctors often recommend a single multi-vitamin/mineral supplement.

**It is nearly impossible for women of child-bearing age to get enough iron in the diet.

*** I.E., cystic fibrosis, cirrhosis, hepatitis, pancreas and gall bladder disease, intestinal disorders, obstructive jaundice.

**** May need multi-vitamin/mineral supplement.

Source: *Runner's World Vitamin Book*, by Virginia DeMoss (Runner's World Books, 1982)

There's one thing you might have noticed as you read through this information: the same foods appeared over and over again. Foods like whole grains, green leafy vegetables, dairy products and fruits supply not only one but a host of vitamins and minerals. This is your cue. When planning your diet, include those vitamin- and mineral-rich foods in your meals all the time.

If, after you've made an effort to use vitamin-laden foods in your meals, you still feel like you want to check into including vitamin and mineral supplements in your diet, it's best to see a nutritionist who can analyze your diet and recommend the supplements that you need. Don't just start taking them without first doing a little research; your body just might not need the ones you choose for it, however well-meaning you might be.

COOKING NUTRITIOUSLY AND DELICIOUSLY

How you cook that food of yours is almost as important to your health and nutrition as the food itself. All cooking, to various degrees, depending on the method used, destroys nutrients, and sometimes the taste of foods. But eating nutritiously does not mean sacrificing great taste. These cooking and preparation suggestions will help you make the most of your food choices — to meet your body's nutritional needs and to please your taste buds as well.

Vegetables

• As mentioned earlier, don't boil! Steam vegetables in just enough water to keep them from burning. Use a tight-fitting lid on your pot so that all of the nutrients will be retained.

• Use the water from your steaming as a gravy for meats or potatoes. Thicken with a little arrowroot if desired.

• Bake or steam potatoes in their skins; don't peel those skins off! The skins are full of vitamins and minerals, and they taste good, too.

• Prepare your salad greens, celery, radishes and other "rabbit food" in bulk. Refrigerate in tight-sealing plastic containers, and then just remove the portion you need at meal time.

• Cut down on the oil in your salad dressings. A dressing of vinegar, lemon juice, spices and a little yogurt tastes great with crisp greens.

• Avoid that salt shaker. Salt hides the natural taste of vegetables. Use lemon juice, herbs and spices instead.

• Combine your vegetables for a great taste medley.

Fruits

• Enhance a fruit's natural flavor with spices like mint, ginger, cinnamon or nutmeg.

• Instead of using sugar as a sweetener, use natural fruit juices.

• Avoid canned fruits packed in heavy syrup; if you can't, rinse the syrup from the fruit with water.

• For a refreshing change, make a fruit salad. You can use just about any fruit you like. If you like creamy salad, moisten with plain yogurt to retain the natural taste of the fruit.

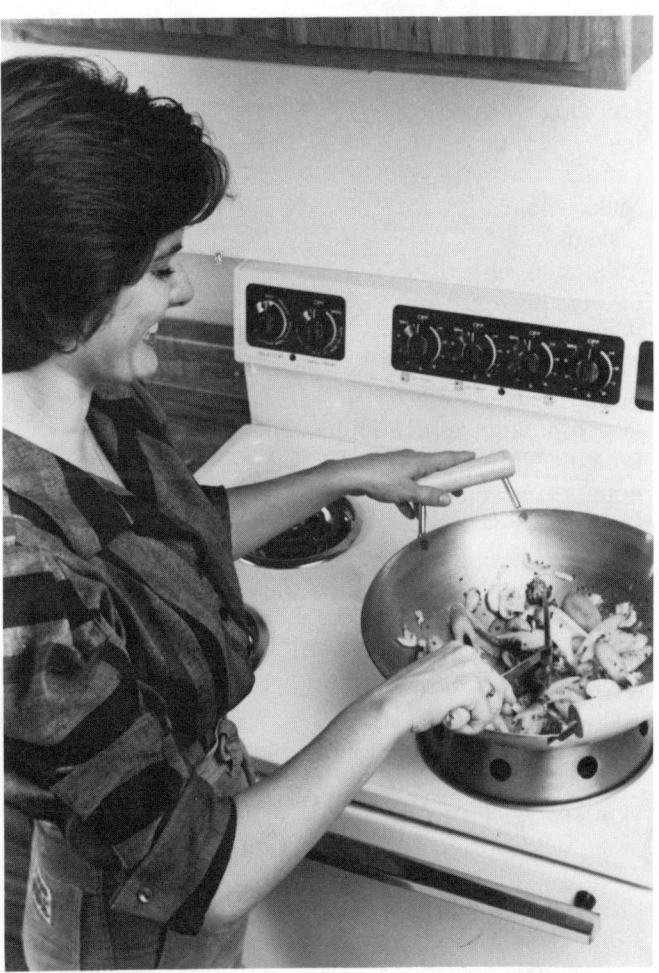

A wok is a great cooking utensil for fresh vegetables.

Counting Your Calories

ITEM	AMOUNT	CALORIES
Apple	2½ inch diameter	70
Bacon, broiled or fried	2 thin slices	60
	2 medium slices	90
Banana	6 × 1½ inches	80
Beef Stew — homemade with lean beef	1 cup	210
Beer	12-ounce can	150
Bread, white	1 slice	75
Butter or margarine	1 pat	50
Carrot	5½ × 1 inches	20
Cauliflower	½ cup of flower buds	10
Cake, chocolate, with chocolate icing	2-inch sector of round layer cake	345
Candy, hard	1 ounce	110
Cheese, American or Swiss	1 ounce	105
Chicken, fried	1 whole leg	225
Chocolate, milk, sweetened	1-ounce bar	150
Cola	12-ounce can	145
Cookies, plain and assorted	1 3-inch	120
Corn-on-the-cob	5-inch ear	70
Corn Flakes	1 cup	95
Eggs, fried in fat	1 large	100
soft or hard boiled	1 large	80
French Fries	10 pieces	155
Ham	3 ounces	245
Hamburger with roll	2-ounce patty	265
Hot Dog with roll	1 average	245
Ice Cream, plain	½ cup	145
Lettuce	2 large leaves	10
Milk, whole	1 cup	160
skim	1 cup	90
Milkshake, chocolate	12 ounces	520
Orange juice, frozen	½ cup	55
Peanut Butter	1 tablespoon	95
Pie, apple	1/7 of 9-inch pie	345
Pizza, plain, cheese	5½ inch sector	185
Popcorn, large kernel popped with oil and salt	1 cup	40
Potato Chips	10 medium	115
Potatoes, baked	5-ounce potato	90
Rice, cooked	¾ cup	140
Salad Dressing, commercial type, Thousand Island	1 tablespoon	80
Spaghetti, with tomato sauce and cheese	¾ cup	195
Strawberries	½ cup	30
Steak, broiled without bone	3 ounces	330
Sugar, white or brown	1 teaspoon	15
Tomato Juice	½ cup	20
Tuna Fish, canned in oil and drained	3 ounces	170
Wine, table	6-ounce glass	150
Whiskey — 80 proof	1½ ounce jigger	95

Source: Home and Garden Bulletin No. 153, U.S. Department of Agriculture, Prepared by Consumer Food Economics Research Division.

Grains and Cereals

- Prepare your cereals without sugar or fat; use skim milk to eliminate fat, and cut up some fresh fruit (bananas, strawberries, blueberries, peaches) instead of using presweetened cereal, or sugar.

- Avoid all the fattening sauces on pasta; it's not the pasta that's fattening, it's the sauce. Enjoy pasta with fresh grated cheese or fresh tomato sauce instead.

- Vary your bread grains. Try a bread made with a number of different grains like rye and millet or a combination of several. Don't stick just to whole wheat.

- It's the butter on the toast that's the killer, not the jam. Spread toast with apple butter or marmalade, and try to skip the butter. You'll hardly notice it's gone.

Dairy Products

- Replace the sour cream and heavy cream in your recipes with yogurt.

- Yogurt can even replace mayonnaise, which is high in saturated fat. Spread it on your bread before you put that sandwich together, and see if it doesn't do the trick.

- Most adults should avoid whole milk. Use low-fat or, better yet, skim milk, in your cooking.

Meats

- Trim off as much fat as possible before cooking meats; remove the skins from chicken pieces.

- Avoid gravies made with a lot of sugar and fat.

- Cook your roasts on a rack so that fat can drip to the bottom of the pan.

- Use water-packed fish. If that's not available, drain the oil from the fish and rinse with very hot water.

- Again, avoid salt. Season instead with herbs and spices.

- Cook meats with dry white or red wines; wine helps burn off calories.

SOME FACTS ABOUT THE SALT OF THE EARTH

Most of us have been shaking salt on our foods since the time we could hold our own forks. A pinch here, a teaspoon there, and that once-blah food seems to taste so much better.

Well, if you really stop and think about it, that food doesn't really taste any better; it just tastes salty. And that salty taste may be doing more to your health than it's doing to your food. More harm, that is.

Those tiny grains of sodium chloride so liberally sprinkled on food are culprits in causing one of America's leading health problems: hypertension, otherwise known as high blood pressure. And high blood pressure is a serious problem both because it can lead to fatal heart diseases and cerebral strokes and because it is sneaky. High blood pressure can go undetected for many years because there are few, if any, apparent symptoms. It can increase in severity, unnoticed, until it causes grave health problems.

So where does salt come into the picture? The sodium in salt is the villain that causes high blood pressure. In the body, one of the main actions of this chemical is to trigger swelling in the walls of the arterioles, the tiny blood vessels that carry fresh, oxygenated blood to the farthest parts of the body.

As the walls of these vessels swell, there is less room for the blood, which is being pumped by the heart at a constant rate, to squeeze through. Blood keeps thudding into the swollen arteries, backs up and causes high blood pressure. In addition to swelling the arterioles, salt causes retention of body fluids, which results in more volume of blood and further raises the blood pressure. This in turn strains the heart.

This noxious effect of salt on the body is cumulative. That means that the salt you ate on food as a small child has already had an effect on your system, and the problem increases with further use.

So what can be done to alleviate the problem? Get rid of the salt shaker! Contrary to popular belief, there are only three tastes that the tongue picks up naturally: sweet, sour and bitter. We pick up the taste of salt early on because of the high amount of salt in baby foods and the foods we eat as a child.

And food does taste good without it. Minus the salt, food tastes fresh and delicate, undisguised by this seasoning that often reduces the varied flavors in food to a uniform sharpness. Abstaining from the use of salt in cooking and seasoning, and avoiding processed foods that contain lots of salt is important in the fight against high blood pressure. And even if you don't have high blood pressure, it's a great preventive health measure and a good way to find out how food really tastes. You might even find that you prefer food enhanced by the natural flavors of herbs and spices instead of blanketed by one taste — salt.

But because your taste buds are used to seasoning, they need a tang of something exciting. Here are some ways to help you enjoy the flavor of natural foods without using salt:

• Use lemon and lime wedges. These tart fruits are just about sodium-free and make food taste great. As a salt substitute, try a squeeze of lemon or lime juice. It has a sharp, fragrant flavor that makes up for the lack of salt.

• Delve into the world of herbs and spices. They add a varied taste interest to food. Use individually or combine.

• Put the salt shaker in the cupboard for a while. When recipes call for salt, avoid it.

• Read labels on food products. Most canned vegetables and many processed foods are high in sodium. Words on labels to beware of: salt, brine, monosodium glutamate, sodium benzoate, sodium bicarbonate, sodium sulfite, sodium hydroxide, sodium cyclamate.

• Homemade salad dressings of vinegar and vegetable oil contain little sodium, but bottled dressings and mayonnaise may be high in sodium. Check labels.

• As mentioned earlier, use only fresh meats. Processed meats are laden with sodium and other unwanted substances.

LEARN TO DO IT YOURSELF

A very good friend of mine eats an absolutely atrocious diet. Nothing but junk, most often procured from the fast-food restaurants around the corner from her house. Wendy's double-deckers, 7-11 burritos and Slurpees — not the healthiest of food, but she figures she can rationalize herself out of eating good, balanced meals. "Who has time?" she says. "I work, and I don't even have enough time to go shopping, let alone try to cook."

This is a sore subject between the two of us, because I think that everyone can and should make the time to eat right without a lot of fuss and preparation. It's true; a lot of us don't have the time during the day to plan out elaborate meals, but who says that a good meal has to be elaborate? Here are a few tips that might help you make nutritious meals — easy — at home.

— Keep your cupboard well-stocked with staples that won't spoil easily. Some things you might want to have around include brown rice, pasta, vegetable or safflower oil, flour, bouillon, honey, baking soda and powder, canned tomatoes and sauce, beans, evaporated milk, cream of mushroom, celery or potato soups, and tuna.

— The same goes for your fridge. Things that should be on call in your refrigerator are eggs, cheese, milk, celery and carrots, butter or margarine. Your freezer can be a good storage place, too. Keep your breads here; they will stay fresher. Tortillas are good to have on hand as well as plenty of chicken pieces and some frozen vegetables, sans all the cream and butter sauces.

— Spices can help turn otherwise boring meals into real taste treats, and they can dissolve your need for lots of salt. Garlic, cinnamon, onion powder, parsley, curry powder, celery seed, marjoram, basil and oregano all help to bring out the flavor of home-cooked foods.

— Take the time at least once a week to plan your weekly menus. It sounds like a pain in the rear, but it will really pay off during the middle of that hectic week.

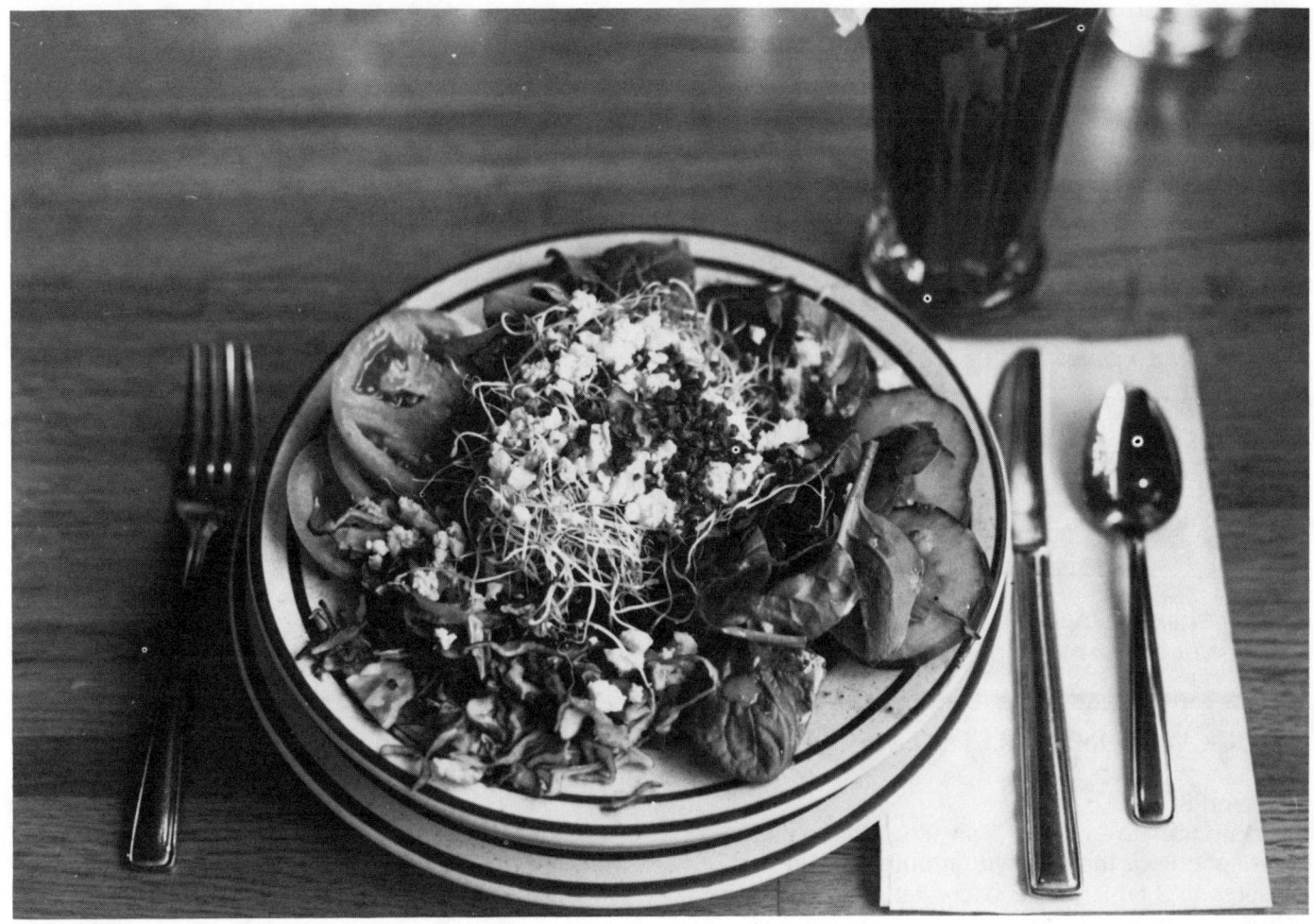

A wholesome salad and drink at lunch provide a well-balanced meal.

— Then make a list of what you need for each of those dinners so that when you go to the market, you know exactly what you need. You won't be forgetting anything important, and you won't fill your cart with a bunch of junk, either.

— Try to do your shopping once each week rather than taking a trip to the grocery store once a month and stocking up for a year. You'll find that you'll buy only what you need, and once you get into the habit, shopping every Monday or Tuesday night will become second nature. By the way, I've found Monday night to be the absolute best time to shop. Mom and the kids are at home, and not in the store; shopping can actually be a pleasurable experience at night.

— If you haven't already, invest in a slow-cooker. Slow-cookers are real time-savers, and they usually make up enough food to feed you and yours for several days. Just remember to add some of your vegetables just before you serve so that they will be crisp.

— Soups are another delicious way to get a good meal. And if you make enough, a good, hearty soup can last you all week.

— Short on time? Make a meal of a salad. Salads don't have to be skimpy, little appetizers. Toss in some water-packed tuna or fresh, baby shrimp with your lettuce, and be sure to add lots of crisp, fresh veggies. Top with a little grated cheese and herbal vinaigrette dressing, serve with hot bread, and you've got a great meal. And it only took you fifteen minutes to prepare. The variations with salads are endless; here's your chance to be creative.

— A lot of those trips to the diner down the street take place at lunchtime, and one way to avoid that is to pack your lunch. Brown-bagging it doesn't have to be boring; be ingenious.

Include things like yogurt, roasted nuts, fresh fruit and trail mix for snacking. And really be creative with your sandwiches: Use different kinds of breads like rye, sourdough French, date-nut or banana-nut, bagels, onion rolls or pocket bread.

— If sandwiches don't ring your bell, take some of yesterday's leftovers with you for lunch. Homemade soup stays nice and hot in a Thermos, and saves lots of money.

— Pack that lunch the night before so you won't have to worry about doing it early in the morning. Keep it in the refrigerator; that way it will be nice and fresh by the time lunch rolls around.

— Feel like something substantial for dinner, but just don't want to spend two hours cooking? Try steaming your meats. (Make sure that you take the meat out of the freezer before you leave in the morning, so you won't have an excuse to hit a fast-food restaurant.) Just place your chicken or pork in a shallow pan, fill with a quarter-inch of water, spice as you like, cover with aluminum foil and pop it in the oven for twenty-five minutes. Voila! Your meat is ready to eat, and nice and juicy to boot. Steaming your meat doesn't dry it out like frying or broiling.

No-Nonsense Recipes

Here are some great ideas for healthy, nutritious breakfast, dinner and lunch foods you can whip up in a jiffy.

CHUCK WAGON SKILLET STEAK

Have on hand:
   1 cup tomato sauce or 1 jar spaghetti sauce
Dredge in flour then brown on both sides in hot skillet with 2 tablespoons bacon fat or oil:
   1½ pound chuck steak cut in fourths
Add to skillet (sliding under steak):
   2 or 3 potatoes, sliced thin
   2 or 3 carrots, sliced thin
   1 can beef broth (10½ ounces)
   1 cup tomato sauce or prepared spaghetti sauce
   ½ cup red wine
   1 teaspoon each: basil, oregano, paprika
   1 tablespoon miso thinned in 1 tablespoon vinegar
Cover and simmer 1 hour, mixing once or twice to rearrange veggies. Add more wine if too dry.

BEER BARBEQUE SAUCE

Combine and use for basting barbecued chicken, ribs, chops or burgers:
   1 cup catsup
   1 cup beer
   ¼ cup each: lemon juice, soy sauce
   2 tablespoons honey
   ½ teaspoon garlic granules or 2–4 cloves garlic, mashed
   2 teaspoons each: chili powder, cumin, dill weed
   1 teaspoon dry mustard powder

REGULAR TOSTADAS

In shallow skillet and 3 inches of very hot oil, fry 60 seconds or until crisp:
   corn or wheat tortillas, as needed to serve
Warm in small saucepans:
   frijoles or use canned refried beans
   shredded burrito beef
Arrange in small bowls or large platter:
   shredded cheese
   diced tomatoes
   shredded lettuce and/or spinach
   minced scallions
   alfalfa sprouts
   sour cream, or yogurt and/or 1 cup yogurt plus 1
      avocado, mashed
   mild taco sauce or green tomatillo sauce
   browned, ground sausage meat, minced
      (optional)
   sliced black or green olives (optional)
   slivered red or green bell pepper (optional)
Arrange all on serving table, and see the many combinations that result from this help-yourself free-for-all.

SUNSET AND VINE SUMMER SALAD

To make Hollywood dressing combine in cruet:
   1 cup yogurt
   2 tablespoons honey or date sugar
   1 tablespoon lemon or lime juice
   blue cheese crumbled to taste
   1 tablespoon toasted sesame seeds or gomasio
      (optional)
Combine in salad bowl:
   1 large bunch romaine lettuce to equal 1 quart
   8 large radishes, quartered
   1 bunch scallions, diced
   4 chopped dates
   ¼ cup raisins
   ¼–½ cup walnut pieces, chopped
   2 tablespoons fresh mint or 1 teaspoon dry
   2 tablespoons parsley, minced
Pour dressing over all and toss.

ORANGE AND CHICKEN SALAD

Brown in 2 tablespoons butter:
    ¼ cup slivered almonds
To make dressing, combine and mix:
    ½ cup cream cheese, softened
    1 teaspoon grated orange peel
    ¼ cup orange juice or 1 tablespoon orange juice
      concentrate and 2 tablespoons water
    salt and pepper to taste
Combine in salad bowl:
    1½ cups cooked chicken, chopped
    2 ribs celery, diced
    1 large orange, peeled and cut in small pieces or
    small can mandarin oranges sliced
    browned almonds (above)
Add dressing and toss to coat. Good as a filling for whole-grain rolls or topping for open-faced sandwich.

BEEF BURGUNDY

Brown in bacon fat or oil:
    2 pounds chuck or stew beef, cubed
Combine in crock pot:
    browned beef (above)
    2 onions, chopped
    2–4 cloves garlic, minced
    1 cup beef broth
    1 cup Burgundy
    1 teaspoon each: marjoram, thyme
    salt and pepper, to taste
Cook on low all day.
In the p.m. saute in olive oil, then add to crock pot:
    ½ pound mushrooms, sliced
To make stew more complete add any or all:
    2 tablespoons cornstarch, thinned in a little water
    small can beets
    small can any type beans
    1 package frozen peas or green beans
Turn to high and cook ½ hour longer.
Serve with boiled potatoes and salad. Freeze leftovers.

IRISH FARM STEW POT

Soak overnight in crock pot:
- 3 cups water
- ½ cup barley
- ½ cup split peas

In the a.m. brown in 2 tablespoons oil (or skip if rushed):
- 1 pound stew meat (lamb or pork) cut bite sized and dredged in flour

Combine in crock pot (with soaked barley, peas and soaking liquid):
- browned meat (above)
- 1 large onion, chopped
- 2 leeks, chopped by hand (well-washed)
- 1 large carrot, sliced
- 1 small or ½ medium head cabbage, shredded
- 2 large or 4 small potatoes cut in large chunks
- 1 tablespoon paprika
- ½ teaspoon salt or to taste
- coarsely ground pepper (to taste)

Simmer on low for 8 to 10 hours.
One half hour before serving mix in 2 tablespoons cornstarch thinned with a little white wine and turn pot to high to thicken.

CURRIED EGGS

Saute in 1 tablespoon butter and 1 tablespoon oil:
- 1 small onion, chopped
- 1 tart apple, diced

Mix in and saute 2 minutes:
- 2 tablespoons flour
- 1–2 teaspoons curry powder or to taste
- 1 teaspoon turmeric
- ½ teaspoon ginger

Add, cook and stir until thick:
- 1 cup chicken broth
- 1 cup yogurt

Add:
- ¼ cup raisins
- ¼ cup chopped cashews or peanuts
- ¼ cup coconut

Arrange:
- 4 hard-cooked eggs on 4 English muffin halves

Cover each with:
- ½ cup sauce

If poached eggs are desired, drop 4 eggs into sauce, cover pan and simmer 4 minutes or until eggs are set. Place each egg on toasted English muffin and cover with ½ cup sauce.

BASIC TOMATO SAUCE

Have on hand:
   6-quart pot with lid (use also for stewing 2–3 chickens at once for freezing)
Chop:
   3 large or small onions
   2–4 green or red bell peppers (if available)
   1 small bunch parsley
Grate:
   2 carrots
   1 small or ½ medium cabbage
Dice:
   2 ribs celery
Chop:
   2–4 cups mushrooms
Mince:
   4–8 cloves garlic to taste
Saute all veggies in 4 tablespoons olive oil until limp. Combine sauteed veggies in pot (above) with:
   3 cans tomatoes (1 pound 12 ounces)
   1 12-ounce can tomato paste
   1½ cups red wine
   ⅓ cup miso thinned with ⅓ cup water
   2 tablespoons molasses
   1 tablespoon basil
   ½ teaspoon coarsely ground pepper
   ½ teaspoon salt
   2 bay leaves
(Note: for variety add):
   2 tablespoons hoisin sauce
Makes 4 quarts
To freeze: pack in a variety of containers ranging in size from 1 cup to 1 quart.

HUEVOS RANCHEROS

Have on hand:
   1½ cups basic tomato sauce
   4 tortillas
Heat in skillet:
   basic tomato sauce (above)
   4 tablespoons mild green chilies, diced or to taste
Add and stir to melt:
   1 cup sharp cheddar cheese
Drop in gently:
   4–6 eggs
Cover and cook until eggs are set. Serve eggs and sauce over warmed tortillas.
Note: To warm tortillas, wrap in foil and heat at 350 degrees for 10 minutes.

ONE-STEP RIGATONI BAKE

Arrange in greased casserole with pasta (uncooked) on bottom:
    2 cups rigatoni or thick whole wheat shells or spiral noodles

    ½ pack (3 tablespoons) dried onion soup mix
    1½ cups water
    ½ to 1 pound lean ground beef, crumbled
Any or all:
    chopped mushrooms, green pepper, onion, celery
    salt and pepper to taste
Top with:
    8-ounce can tomato sauce
    ⅓ cup parmesan cheese
Cover and bake at 350 degrees for 50 minutes. Uncover and bake 10 minutes.

HOMESTYLE APPLY CRUMBLE

Preheat oven: 350 degrees
Combine and put in greased 8-inch-square pan:
    8 tart apples, cut in thin wedges
    ½ cup brown sugar
    ¼ cup honey
    2 tablespoons wheat flour
    ¼ cup apple or orange juice
    ½ cup raisins or chopped dates
    ½ teaspoon each: allspice, ginger
    1 teaspoon cinnamon
    ¼ teaspoon salt
Optional:
    Add coarsely chopped walnuts
Top apple mix with:
Combine:
    ½ stick butter or margarine
    1 cup quick-cooking oats
    ½ cup each: whole-wheat flour, wheat germ or
      ⅔ cup whole-wheat pancake mix
    ½ cup brown sugar
    1 teaspoon each: ginger, coriander
    ¼ teaspoon salt or 1 tablespoon gomasio
Press topping onto apples. Bake at 350 degrees for 40–50 minutes.

HAMBURGER CASSEROLE

Have on hand:
 1 pack frozen limas, thawed
 1 pack frozen corn, thawed
Briefly stir-fry together:
 1 pound hamburger
 1 onion, chopped
In bowl squeeze with hands (to crush and mix):
 canned tomatoes (1 pound 12 ounces)
 2–4 teaspoons curry powder or to taste
 2 tablespoons miso (optional — if available)
Slice very thin:
 2 large potatoes
 2 green peppers (if available)
Arrange in layers until all is used, sprinkling each with flour (⅓ cup in all), salt and pepper as follows:
1) hamburger mix, 2) potatoes, 3) corn and 4) limas.
Pour tomatoes over all.
Cook on low 8 to 10 hours. One hour before serving, cover with grated cheddar cheese.

SUMMER FRUIT AND CHICKEN SALAD

Combine:
 2 cups cooked chicken, chopped
 2 cups peaches and/or nectarines, sliced
 2 ribs of celery, diced
 ½ cup sour cream or (low-calorie) yogurt
 2 teaspoons soy sauce
 1 teaspoon honey
 1 tablespoon crystalized ginger or dried
  pineapple, chopped
 1 bunch watercress, chopped
Spread on whole-grain bread. Sprinkle with sunflower seeds.

EGGS A LA WELSH RAREBIT

Warm in saucepan:
 3 tablespoons milk
Stir in and melt:
 1 cup sharp cheddar cheese, grated
 2 tablespoons butter
 ¼ teaspoon salt
 coursely ground pepper to taste
 1 teaspoon Dijon-type mustard.
Poach:
 2–4 eggs
Toast:
 2–4 English muffin halves
Top muffins with eggs and cover with cheese sauce. Makes breakfast for two.

TOUTE LES CHOSES PORK POT

Soak in crock pot overnight in enough water to cover by 1 inch:
   1 cup white beans
In a.m. add to pot:
   1 cup white wine
   1 teaspoon rosemary leaves
   ½ teaspoon marjoram
   fresh ground pepper
   1½–2 pounds lean pork, ½-inch cubes
   1 cup or 1 can chicken broth
   ½ teaspoon salt
Slice and add:
   few potatoes
   celery
   carrots and/or parsnips
   1 onion, chopped
Cook on low all day.
In p.m. saute in olive oil and add to pot:
   2 cloves garlic, chopped fine
Combine (blend) and add to pot:
   4 tablespoons flour
   1 cup yogurt
Add to pot:
   1 pack frozen green peas, thawed
   few tomatoes, peeled and sliced
Cook ½ hour longer on high. Freeze leftovers.

POACHED EGGS WITH SOUPY SAUCE

Heat to simmer
   1 can condensed tomato or mushroom soup
     (10½ ounces)
   ¼ cup milk
Stir in and melt:
   1 cup shredded cheddar cheese
Drop in gently:
   4 eggs
Cover pan and simmer 4 minutes or until eggs are set. Serve on whole-grain bread, toasted or English muffins. Topped with sprouts or avocado slices.

LIFE SAVER WAKE-UP SHAKE

Combine in blender and whip until smooth:
   1 cup yogurt
   1 ripe banana
   1 egg yolk
   2 tablespoons brewer's yeast
   1 heaping tablespoon carob powder
   1 heaping tablespoon protein powder
   splash of juice, milk or water to thin

LENTIL SOUP WITH HAM

Soak in water to cover overnight:
    1 cup lentils
In a.m. put in crock pot:
soaked lentils
    4 cups water
    1 onion, chopped
    1 smoked ham shank
Any or all:
    Diced carrots, celery, turnip, parsnip; shredded
      chard, kale, collards or cabbage
    1 teaspoon each: marjoram, thyme, salt, cumin,
      basil
    freshly ground pepper to taste
Cook on low 8 to 10 hours before serving, remove ham shank, strip off meat and dice. Return ham to soup.

HAMBURGER AND GREEN VEGETABLE STIR-FRY

To make sauce, combine:
    1 can beef broth (10½ ounces)
    1 tablespoon cornstarch (thinned with a little
      broth)
    2 tablespoons soy sauce
    2 tablespoons sherry or sake
    1 heaping tablespoon miso
    1 teaspoon molasses
In hot wok stir-fry 5 minutes:
    1 pound lean ground beef
    1 large onion, chopped
    2 cloves garlic, minced
    ½-inch piece of ginger, finely chopped
    1 green or red bell pepper coarsely chopped
Add and stir-fry a few minutes:
    1 bunch broccoli in flowerets
    ¼ pound mushrooms, sliced (optional)
    few carrots, in matchsticks (optional)
Add 2 tablespoons water, lower heat to medium, cover and steam 5 minutes:
Add, cover and steam five minutes:
    prepared sauce (above)
    1 bunch spinach, chopped or 1 pack frozen
      spinach, thawed
Serve immediately with brown rice, udon, or oriental noodles.

SPANISH BROWN RICE

To use brown rice:
Bring to boil, lower heat, cover and simmer ½ hour:
- 1 cup brown rice
- 1 cup beef broth
- 1 cup water

Steam covered in a little water 5 minutes, then turn up heat and brown:
- 8 link sausages

Remove sausages, cool and slice. Saute in same pan with drippings:
- 1 large onion, chopped
- 1–3 green peppers, chopped
- 2–3 cloves garlic, mashed

Add to veggies and simmer 5 minutes:
- 2 large or 4 small tomatoes, skinned and chopped (see note)
- ¼ cup parsley
- 1 teaspoon each: oregano, cumin
- salt and cayenne to taste

Note: to skin tomatoes, plunge in boiling water 1 minute to loosen skins.

Combine tomato sauce plus sausage in greased 2½-quart casserole and mix in:
- precooked brown rice (above) plus cooking liquid or 1 cup quick brown rice plus 1⅓ cup beef broth

Cover and bake at 350 degrees for 35 minutes.

SWEET AND SOUR MEATBALLS

Preheat: 450 degrees
Combine and shape into balls:
- 2 pounds ground beef
- 4 slices dry bread
- 1 egg
- 1 tablespoon catsup
- 1 small onion, chopped fine
- 1 tablespoon milk or yogurt
- salt and pepper to taste

Bake meatballs in baking pan at 450 degrees for 15 minutes. Then turn heat to 350 degrees. Cover meatballs with sauce and continue baking for 45 minutes.

To make sauce, combine:
- 2 cans condensed tomato soup
- 4 tablespoons vinegar
- 4 tablespoons brown sugar

These recipes are excerpted from the *Runner's World No Time To Cook Cookbook* by Diana Frank (Runner's World Books, 1981).

EAT RIGHT — AT THE RIGHT TIME

An old roommate of mine had a very demanding job, and consequently, she always maintained that she never had any time to eat. She passed up breakfast every morning and, lived on snacks from the vending machines and catering trucks while she was at work. By the time she got home each night, she was ravenous, and she would literally "pork out" on anything she could get her hands on. "Bad days" were even worse — even if she wasn't hungry, she would make huge dinners for herself; eating made her feel better, she said.

Another woman I know is overweight and knows that she should cut down on her food intake. Yet, when she is around food, she craves it. She can't even pass up a candy machine without popping in a quarter, and half the time, after she has eaten half of her snack, she begins to feel guilty. "I don't even want this," she says. But she keeps right on munching.

When and why we eat is almost as important to good health and fitness as what we eat. Here are some good eating habits to consider before you pick up your fork and dig in, or before you decide to skip that breakfast of yours:

— Eat when your mind is at ease, if this is possible. We have a tendency to overeat if we are nervous, angry, depressed or worn down. Relax a little before you sit down to eat. You'll feel better, and your digestive system will work better, too.

— Slow down! For some reason, people feel that they have to race through a meal as though the food will get up and walk off the plate before they have a chance to eat it. It won't. Take your time; chew all of your food thoroughly, and try to put your fork down between bites. The person you are dining with will thank you, because you'll be able to carry on a conversation. And since you'll feel full faster, you won't have to get up for that second or third helping.

— Drink lots of water with your meals. We don't begin to drink all the water that we should (doctors and nutritionists recommend eight glasses per day), and drinking helps to fill you up. It's also an aid to digestion.

— If you aren't all that hungry, just don't eat as much. Chances are that you consume far more food than you need each day, and you don't have someone looking over your shoulder making sure you eat big meals. Or clean your plate. Don't feel bad about not finishing a meal if you can't eat it all, even if you are dining at a fancy restaurant. When you feel full, stop eating; your dinner companions will admire your discipline.

— Try to eat at least three meals a day. Breakfast is a toughy for some people; it means getting up a little bit earlier and taking the time to fix it. But breakfast is an important meal because it sets the tone for your entire day. Do your best to fill up in the morning, even if your meal consists of just a piece of bread and some fruit.

— Another good reason to eat breakfast is so that you won't have to eat an eight-course meal in the evening. Research has indicated that calories are absorbed more slowly at night than during the day, based on the fact that blood circulation slows down while you sleep (the absorption of calories depends upon the action of blood circulation.) Therefore, it is wise to cut down on the number of calories you consume in the evening hours. Try not to eat too much after about 7 p.m. Give your body a chance to rest at night.

After rambling on for this long about eating right, could there possibly be anything else of greater importance? Well, maybe not of greater importance, but certainly of equal worth is exercise. Diet can't work effectively to build you a beautifully fit figure without a little help from you. And that means a little sweat. So let's move on to exercise.

2 EXERCISE

MODIFIED FOR HIGH PERFORMANCE: EXERCISE

Why Exercise?

When I was in high school, hot-rod cars were all the rage with the guys (some things never change). Even my boyfriend was a victim of this disease. He had a '67 Mustang, into which went practically every ounce of his time and effort, not to mention his life's savings. I thought it would stop once he had the car painted. It was really a splendid paint job, "trick" as we called it then.

But the tinkering under the hood didn't stop as I thought it would. In fact, it made him more determined than ever to equip his hot rod with every high-performance part imaginable. New gears, new manifold, headers, a four-barrel carburetor. I finally got fed up, and one day, while we were sitting in his parents' garage amid a flood of grease and car parts, I began to yell at him. "When is it going to stop?" I asked. "When is it going to be 'hot' enough for you?" He smiled and said, "Cath, what good is the paint job if the car doesn't run good?"

Well, I never did agree with him about the car, but he did have a point: What's the use of making something look good on the outside if it doesn't work well on the inside?

Your body operates on much the same principle, or it should, anyway. Obviously, it doesn't need a four-barrel carburetor and high-performance parts, but it does need the same kind of high-performance care. A good diet, of course, is essential to maintaining a proper level of fitness and health, but what happens to that great diet if you don't do anything with your body to make that diet work for you? It's like pouring all kinds of expensive, high-performance fuel into an old, beat-up car that doesn't go more than two miles before it breaks down on you. It's just not worth the investment for the fuel unless the car runs properly. You have to help make that fuel work efficiently in your body, too. And the key to efficiency, of course, is exercise — lots of it.

Getting Off Your Duff

Have you ever caught yourself letting one of these one-line excuses slip when someone invites you to work out together?

- "Oh, I get home so late from work; I just don't have the time."
- "There's the children, you know. What will the children do if I'm off exercising?"
- "I run around all day at work; I think that's plenty of exercise."
- "I hate to exercise. It's just plain too hard."
- "Oh, I'm really not the athletic type."
- "I'm not overweight, and I don't have any other physical problems. Why do I need to exercise?"

What You Should Weigh

Persons with wide shoulders and hips and large wrists and ankles can consider themselves in the "large frame" category. Those with narrow shoulders and hips and small wrists and ankles can consider themselves as having a "small frame." Most people fall in the "medium frame" category. Your estimated ideal weight should not change as you become older.

MEN

Feet & Inches	Small Frame lbs	Medium Frame lbs	Large Frame lbs
5'3"	118	129	141
5'4"	122	133	145
5'5"	126	137	149
5'6"	130	142	155
5'7"	134	147	161
5'8"	139	151	166
5'9"	143	155	170
5'10"	147	159	174
5'11"	150	163	178
6'	154	167	183
6'1"	158	171	188
6'2"	162	175	192
6'3"	165	178	195

WOMEN

Feet & Inches	lbs	lbs	lbs
5'	100	109	118
5'1"	104	112	121
5'2"	107	115	125
5'3"	110	118	128
5'4"	113	122	132
5'5"	116	125	135
5'6"	120	129	139
5'7"	123	132	142
5'8"	126	136	146
5'9"	130	140	151
5'10"	133	144	156
5'11"	137	148	161
6'	141	152	166

Source: The Healthy Approach to Slimming, ©*American Medical Association.*

Don't feel bad. In American society today, you are more the rule than the exception. How far we have come from the days of our ancestors, who ran wildly to escape predators, who climbed trees and hiked for miles in search of food, who used their bodies in every way imaginable just to live from day to day. Not many of us would want to step back in time and fill our ancestors' shoes (or bare feet, rather); the conveniences of modern-day life have made living much less of a grind and, certainly for most, more enjoyable. But that same modern-day living has de-emphasized the importance of exercise. Our ancestors did it without thinking; they had to use their bodies in order to survive. But since we don't have to climb trees for food or flee saber-toothed tigers and attacking enemy tribes, exercise is no longer a necessity. It's an option that many of us opt not to worry about anymore.

That wouldn't be so bad, except that the body needs exercise, not just to look good and feel good, but to function properly at all. We can look around us and see the negative effects of life without exercise: excess weight, diminished muscle tone and strength, decreased flexibility and mobility. It's downright impossible to go through one day without encountering several sagging waistlines, lots of bulging hips and thighs and generally dumpy bodies. Does anyone really want to have a dumpy body? Of course not. But the excuses we make *not* to get in shape make it seem like we all want to be fatties forever.

It's true; most of us do have full and busy days, whether we're saddled with the responsibilities of our home and children, or whether we run our tails off on the job. But if you think about it, you really only need about thirty to forty minutes three or four times a week for a good exercise program. Learn to plan exercise into your day. How about on your lunch hour? Maybe it would be possible to eat that tuna sandwich after your workout. Or why not get up a little bit earlier in the morning? It's tough, but the morning is a beautiful time to exercise, both indoors and out, and a nice morning workout will leave you refreshed and ready to tackle the day. How much television do you watch? Perhaps there's one show you might cut out to make time for some brisk walking or running. There's always time for exercise, if you stop and make the time for it.

A lot of people complain that exercise is not enjoyable. Something is wrong then. Perhaps you have started out too rapidly. The idea behind a good, sensible workout is to start out at a level that is comfortable for you, and proceed to a higher level when your body is prepared. Obviously, a first-time jogger will not be able to go out and win a marathon, but winning marathons is not part of beginning an exercise program.

Don't be discouraged. Your body did not get

out of shape overnight, so don't expect it to perform miracles and get back into shape overnight. Good things take time, as we all know, and getting in shape is one of those good things. And don't ever say that you're not athletic. You don't need to be athletic; you just need to be active.

And being active has a great many benefits:

• Your body will build up greater strength and stamina, with a similar reduction of aches and body pains.

• If you suffer from back problems, exercise might help. Back pain is largely an industrial disease; most often it is caused by our sedentary way of life.

• Even if you feel like you're going to drop at the end of the day, health experts guarantee that some good, vigorous exercise will pep you up. When you stimulate your heart and lungs and body muscles, your energy level correspondingly increases.

• To take that notion a step further, you will probably find that you need less sleep, because the sleep you do get is much more restful.

• Exercise is one of the best ways to reduce the often harmful effects of stress and tension in our lives. It gives us an outlet to vent our frustrations, and it helps to physically reduce the amount of tension in muscles and nerves.

• You will notice that your body coordination improves, and that your movements are executed with more grace and agility.

THE WARMUP

Before you begin any athletic activity, treat your body to a good warmup. The purpose of the warmup is to loosen the joints and muscles avoid injuries, speed up the action of the heart and lungs, and to prepare your body for what's in store. A warmup need not take long — just five to ten minutes.

Always start slowly with your warmup. Relaxed, easy stretching of the neck and shoulder muscles is a good way to begin. Then, gradually increase the intensity of your warmup. You should pay special attention to your lower back and leg muscles, as these are often strained during exercise.

Sometimes a warmup is fun to do to music. Yoga positions and stretches also make good warmup exercises, or you may have improvised favorites of your own. But, remember, even if you are short of time, it is wise to take the extra five minutes to warm up than risk injury.

Neck Roll

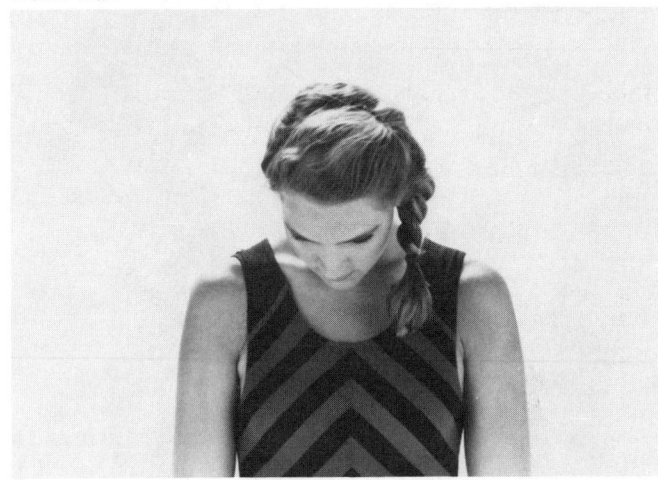

a. *A good warmup is the Neck Roll.*

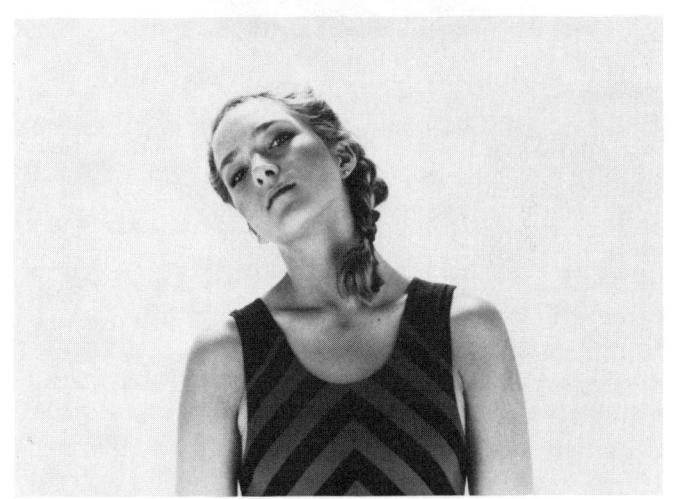

b. *Drop your head to each side and front and back.*

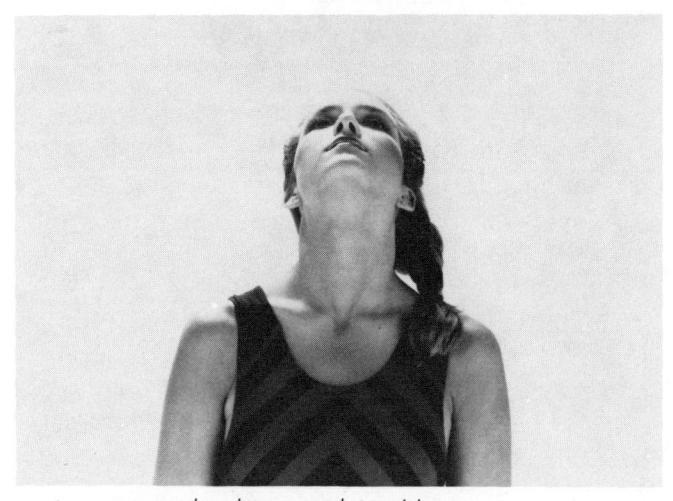

c. *Let your neck relax at each position.*

30 FIGURE MAINTENANCE

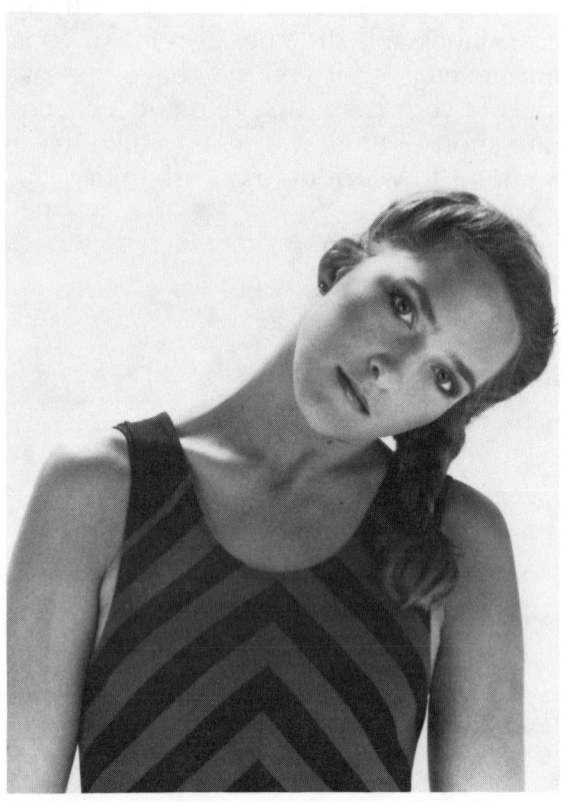

d. *Go slowly and you will increase flexibility.*

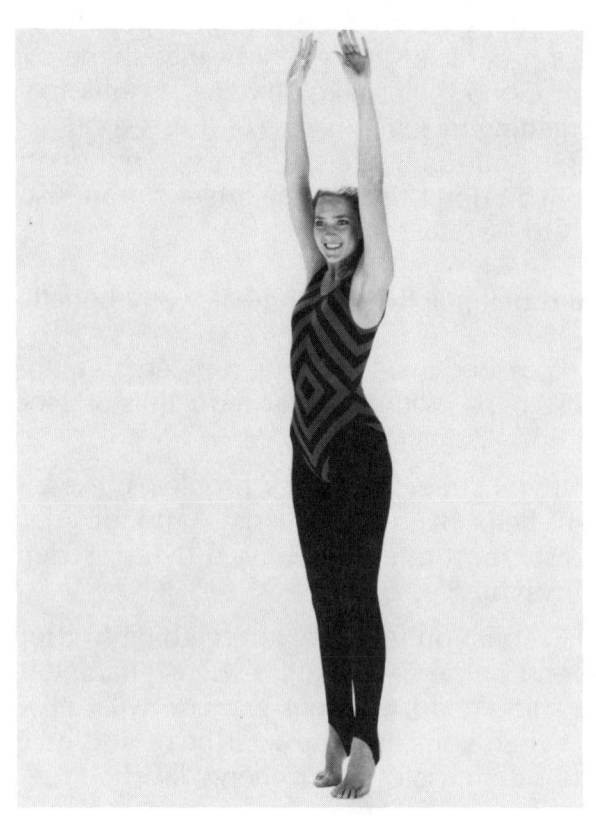

b. *Now reach for the sky, standing on your toes.*

Body Stretch

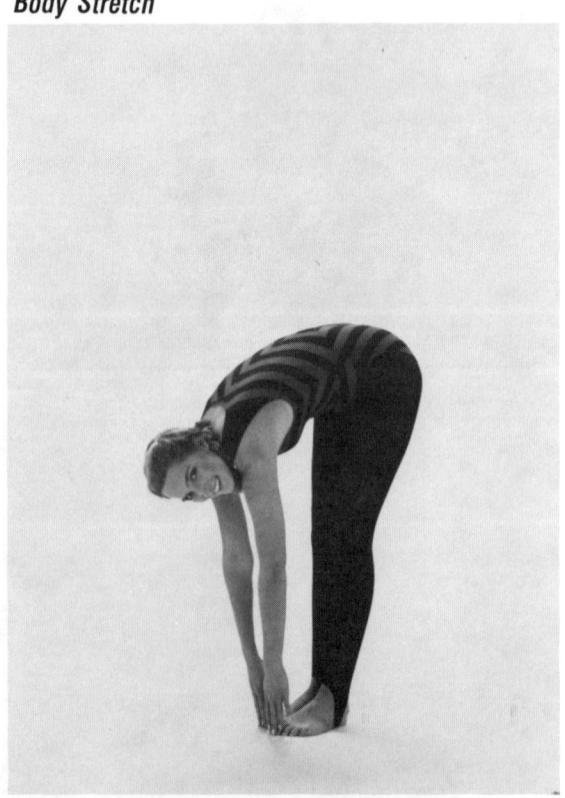

Side Bends

a. *Start the Body Stretch with toes touching feet.*

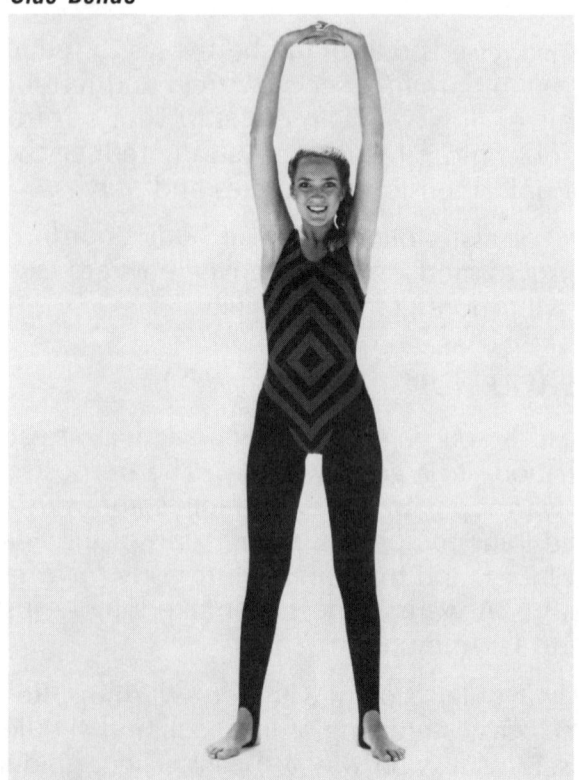

a. *In Side Bends, hold your hands over your head.*

Exercise 31

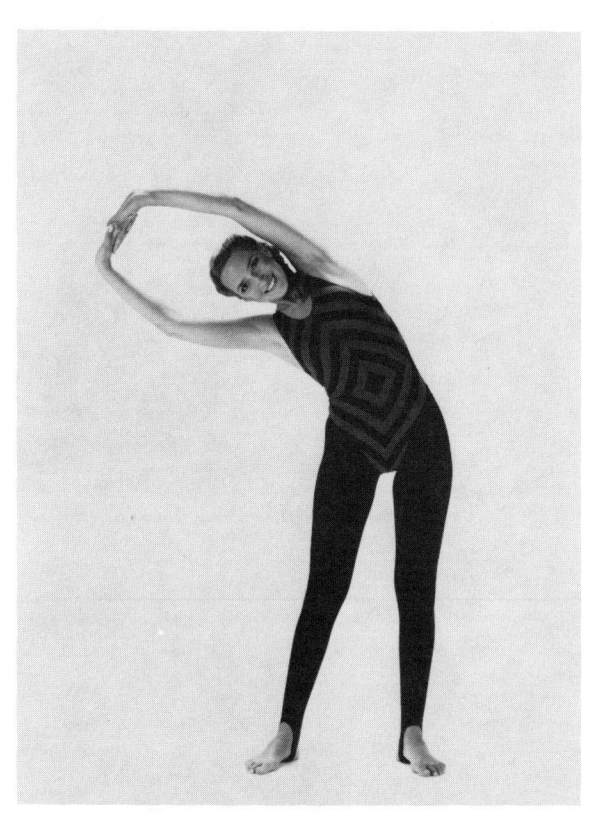

b. *Now, keeping arms and legs straight, bend at the waist to one side.*

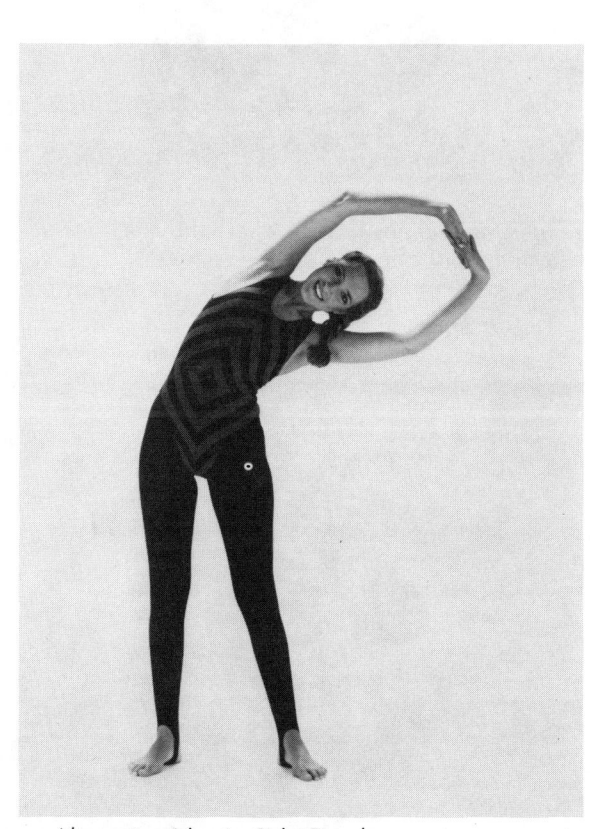

c. *Alternate sides in Side Bends.*

Sprinter's Pose

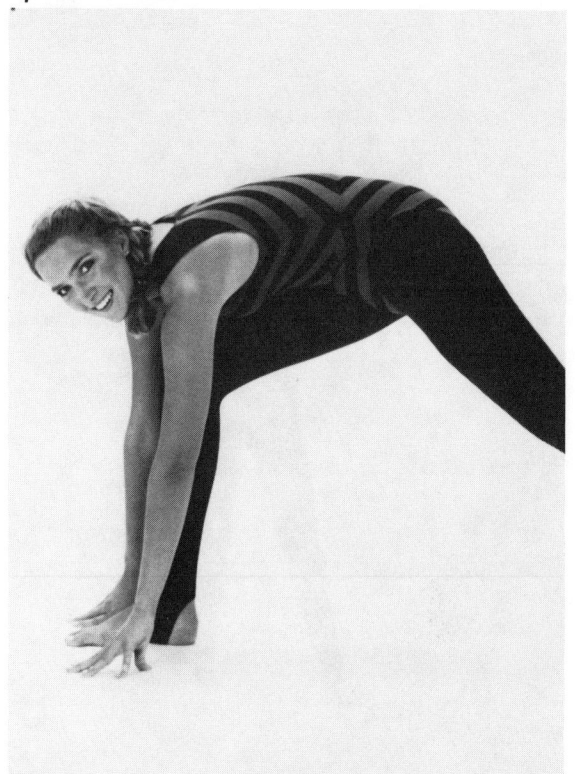

a. *Stretch out one leg in Sprinter's Pose.*

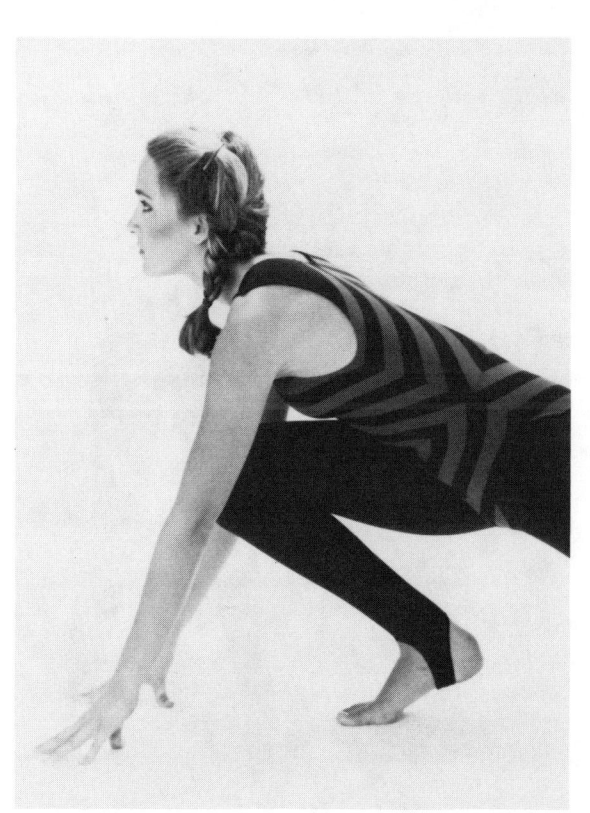

b. *Now arch your back and look up. This stretches the back and stomach muscles.*

FIGURE MAINTENANCE

Toe Touches

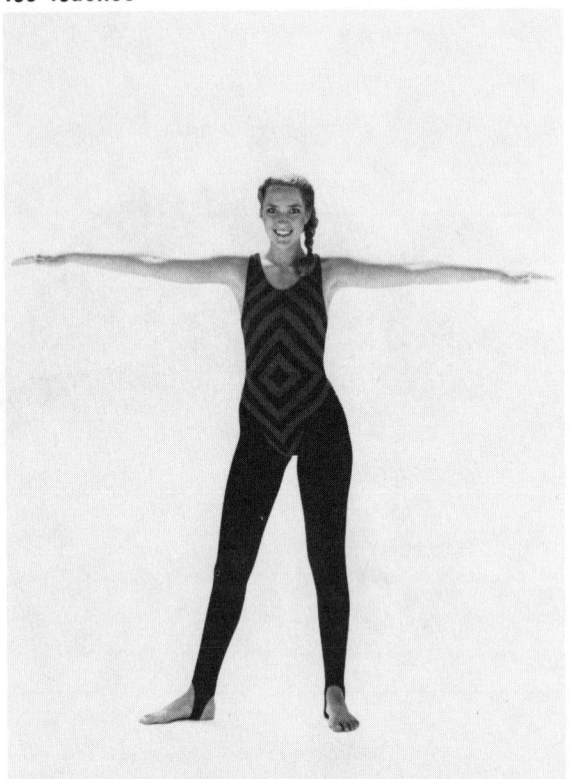

a. Toe Touches increase flexibility in the back and hamstrings.

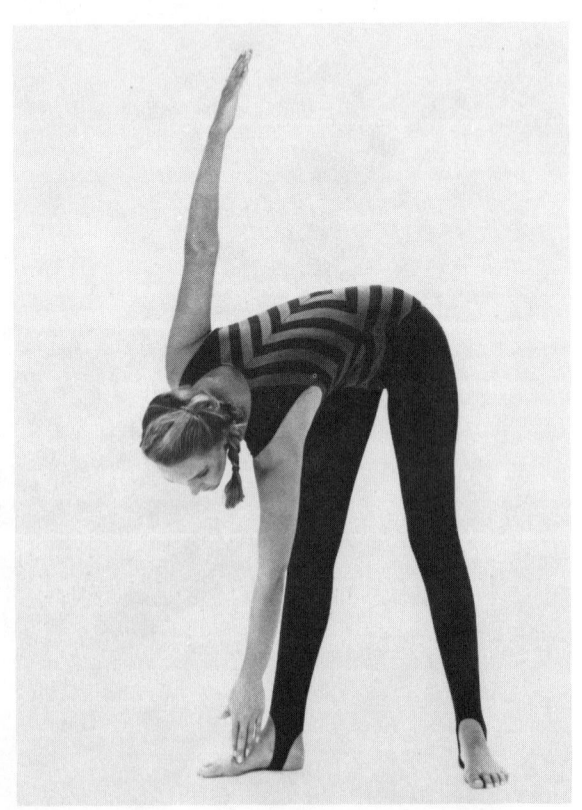

b. Try to touch your toes; if you can't, keep practicing.

Egg Roll

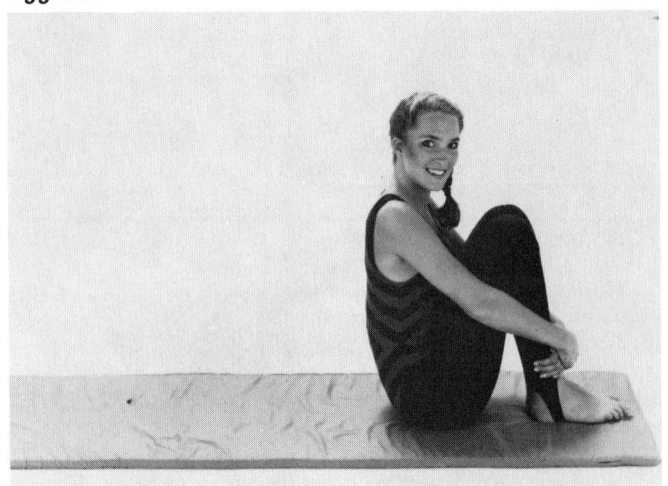

a. Egg Roll is fun to do and relaxes back muscles.

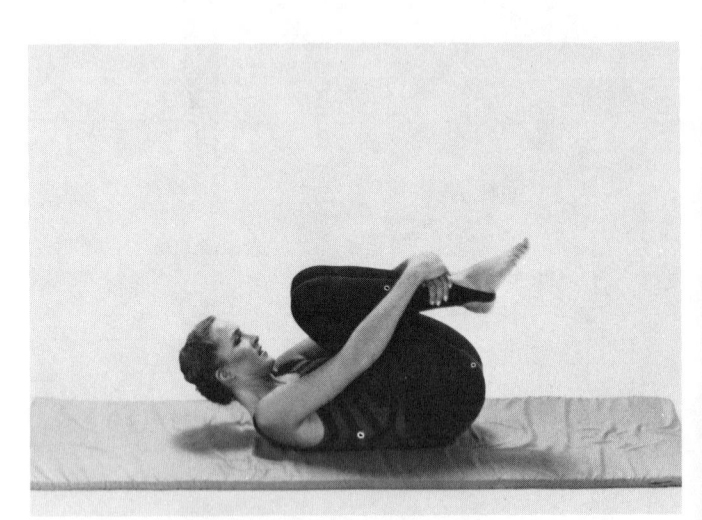

b. Tuck your knees to your chest and roll backward, on a mat or carpet.

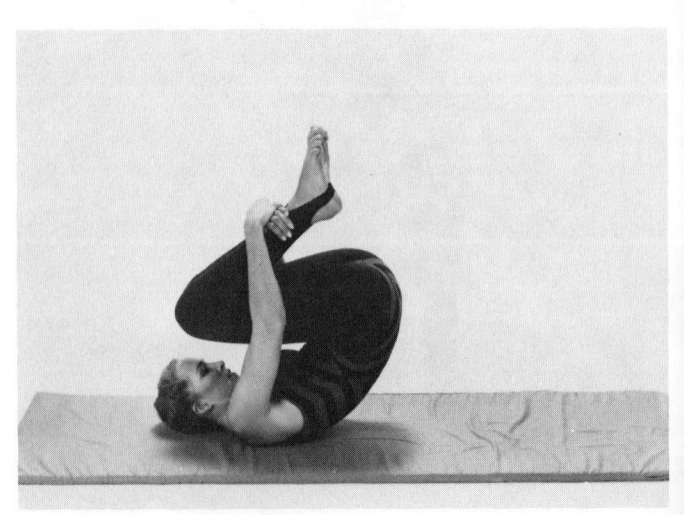

c. Roll all the way back to your head, slowly.

Exercise 33

Kowtow

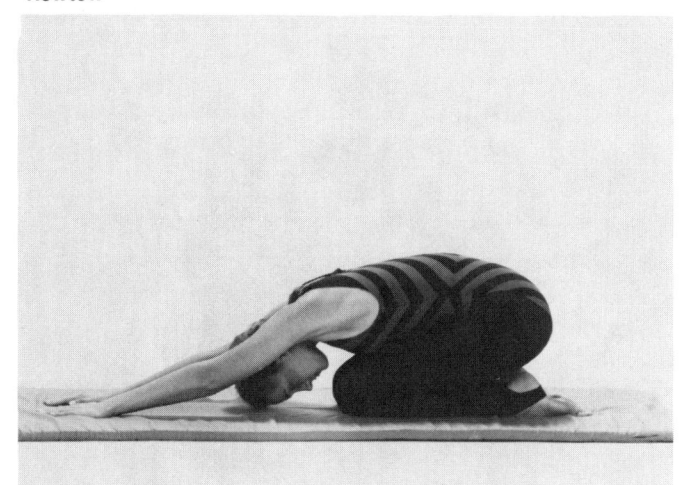

The Kowtow is a great pose for stretching the back, quadriceps, and the arms.

Leg Cross-Over

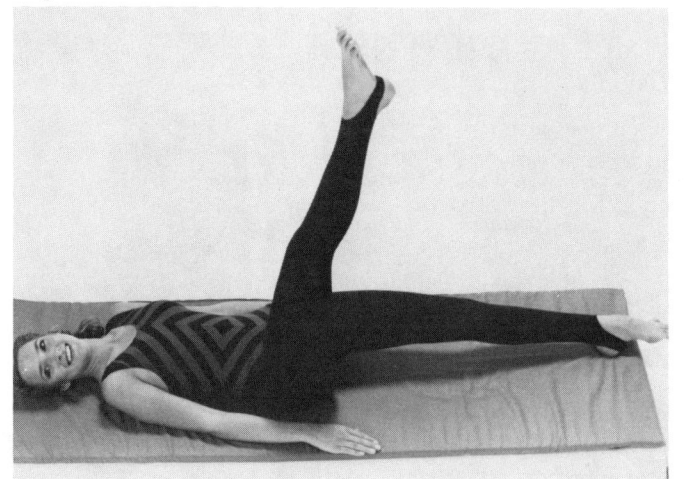

a. Begin the Leg Cross-Over by lifting a leg.

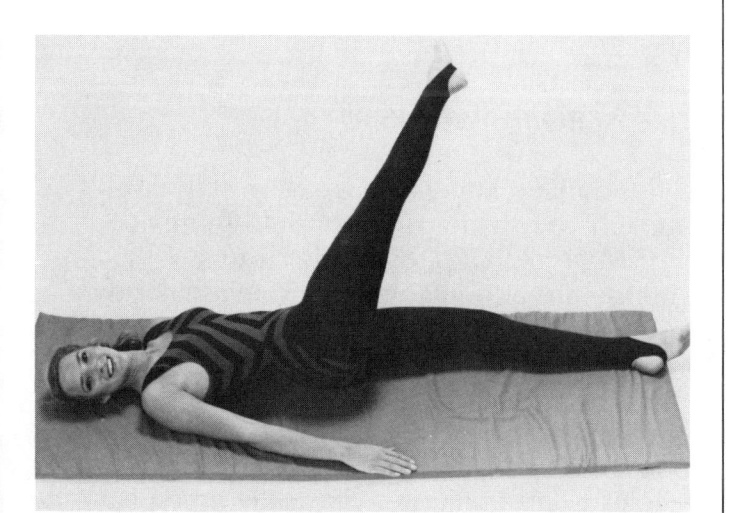

b. Now cross the leg over your resting leg and stretch.

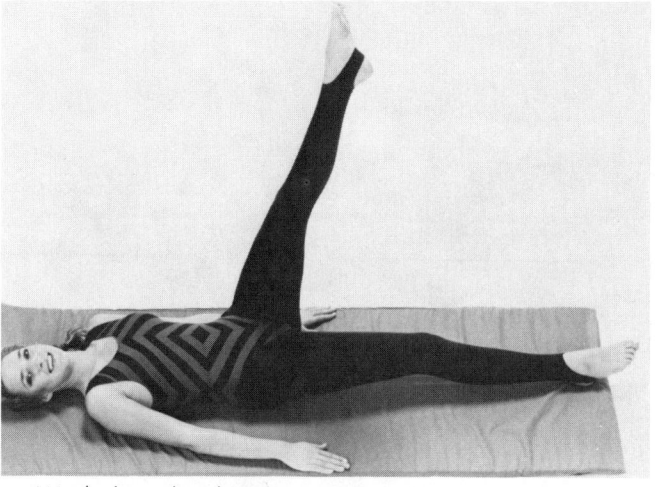

c. Work the other leg the same way.

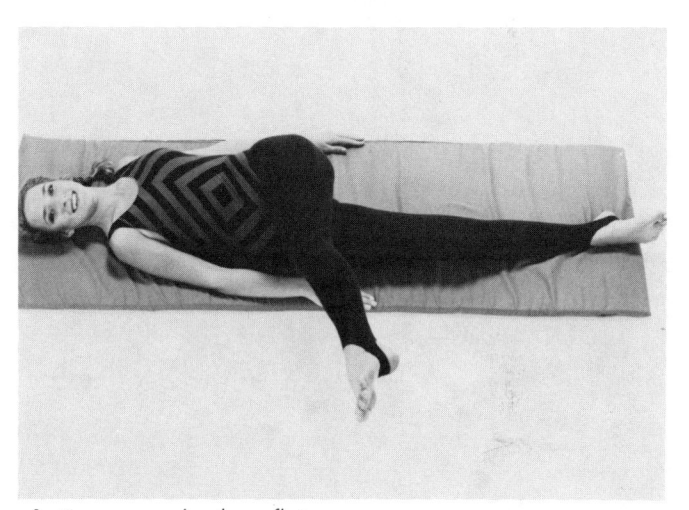

d. Keep your back as flat as you can.

Bent Leg Cross-Over

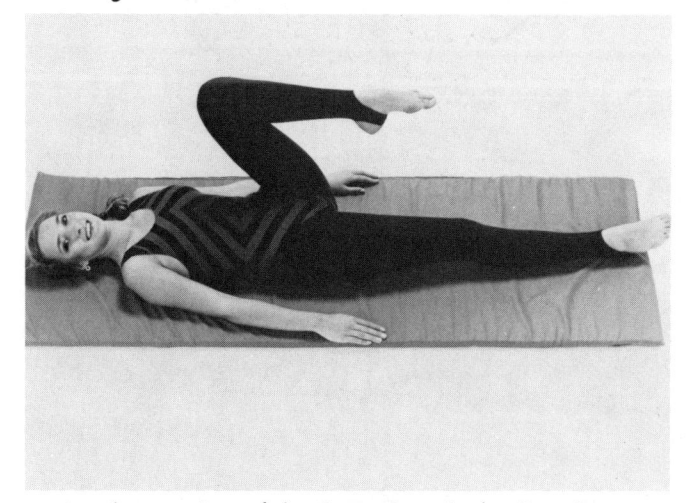

a. Another version of the Cross-Over is the Bent Leg Cross-Over.

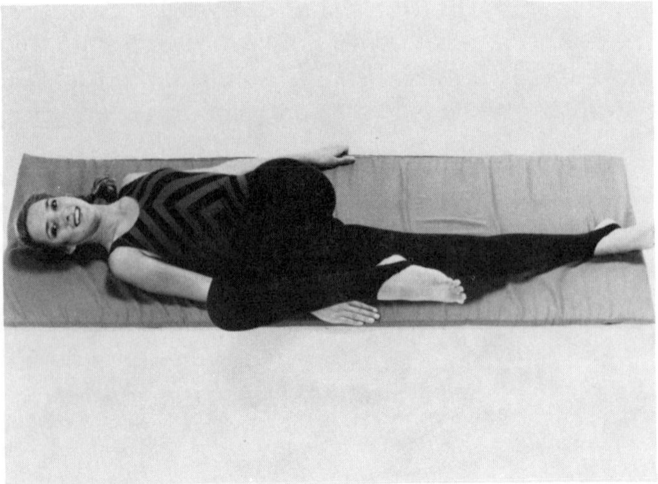

b. *This stretches the hip muscles and increases flexibility in the hip.*

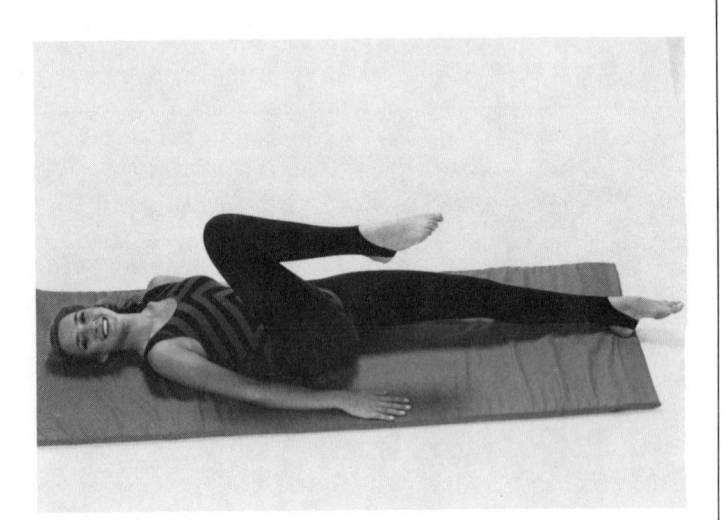

c. *Keep your back as flat as you can.*

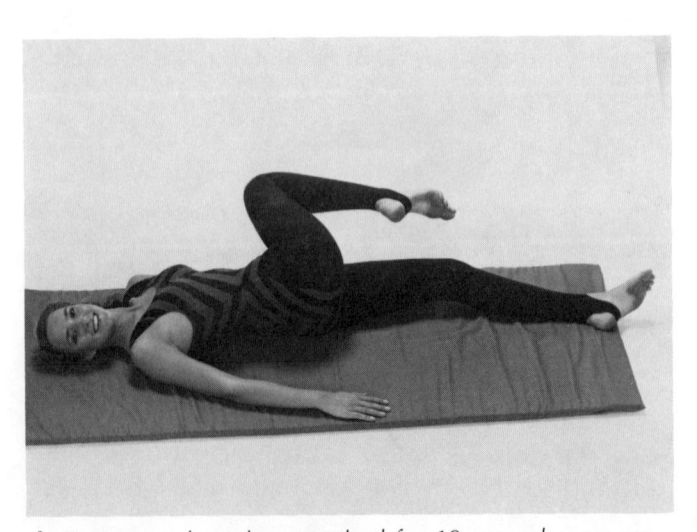

d. *Keep your bent leg stretched for 10 seconds or more.*

Hamstring Stretch

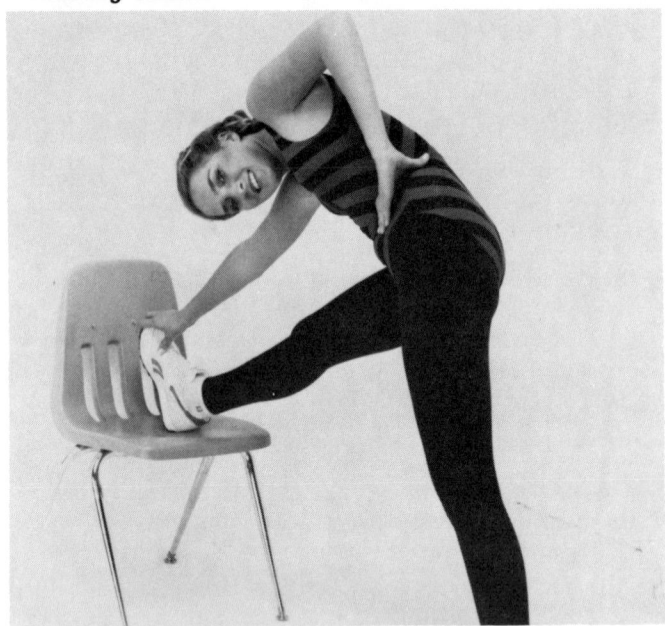

In the Hamstring Stretch, use a chair or ledge.

The Bridge

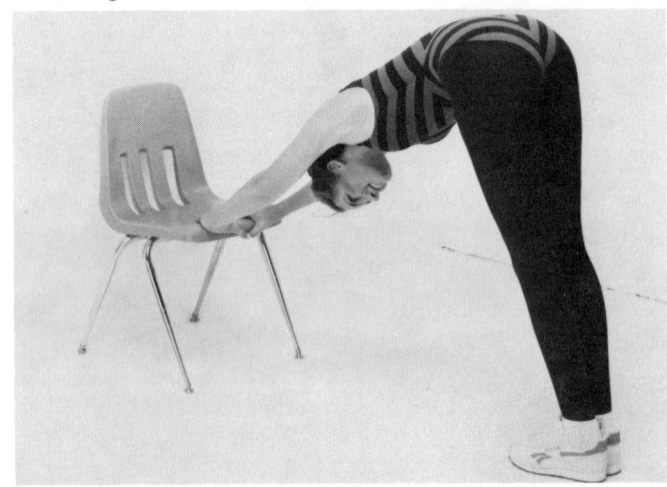

The Bridge calls for keeping the back straight. Stretch your arms.

THE AEROBIC WORKOUT

If the many benefits of exercise still haven't hooked you, perhaps you should think about this: More than half of all the deaths in this country are attributable to cardiovascular dysfunction, commonly referred to as heart disease. Why? Just look at our sedentary lives. We spend most of our days on our butts, eating the wrong kinds of food (but not after reading this book), using machines that do all the real work, smoking and drinking — basically doing damage to our bodies. You may think that all that racing around you do day-to-day is enough, but chances are it's not.

What is the best way to exercise that heart muscle? Glad you asked. There is, and it's called aerobics. Basically, aerobics means with air, more specifically, the oxygen in the air. The muscles in our bodies need oxygen to function, and their demand for oxygen increases dramatically when we work them hard. As you exercise harder, your muscles' need for oxygen goes up, and so does your heart rate. By working those muscles, then, you increase your heart rate, strengthen the heart itself, as well as help your body to burn off excess fat. In essence, the body becomes a more efficient machine.

Put together the two words "aerobic exercise" and you get this: any continuous, steady exercise that demands uninterrupted output from the muscles for at least twelve minutes. Obviously, not all athletic activity offers this type of continuous, high-intensity muscle exercise. A game of golf, for instance, is not sufficient to work the muscles enough to be called aerobic exercise. Nor is baseball when you look at it from this view. Running or cross-country skiing, however, are good aerobic exercises.

The importance of *continuous* and *steady* can't be emphasized enough. Running for five minutes, then stopping, and then running again for another seven minutes will not give as good an aerobic workout as running continuously. But, then again, don't start out working your body too hard. As with your warmup, gradually ease into a program that is comfortable for you. You want to sweat, yes, but you don't want to hurt yourself or become discouraged.

The Aerobic Exercises

Your aerobic workout needn't be boring or unenjoyable, because there are a myriad of different activities that provide aerobic benefits to suit everyone's interests. Here are a few of them:

Walking — There is really no exercise that is as enjoyable, or as easy, as just plain walking. Most of us should walk far more than we do, but since we have become accustomed to driving all over the place, we usually don't use those pups like we should.

Starting out with brisk walking is a good way to begin an exercise program, and it doesn't involve the sweating common to many aerobic exercises. Sometimes, a brisk walk followed by a few minutes of slow jogging can also be tolerated by the beginning exerciser.

If you haven't a walked in a while, leave your car at home and take a stroll to the market for the few things that you need. Or, instead of sitting down for your entire lunch hour, bring a sandwich from home and walk to the park to eat, and bring a friend along.

Minimum time required for aerobic benefit: twenty minutes.

Bicycling — Another activity most of us neglected as soon as we got our hot little hands on a driver's license, bicycling has regained popularity as a pastime and as a viable exercise activity.

When you are considering bicycling as an aerobic activity, take into account only the time spent pedaling. If you are on a long downhill stretch, put your bike into high gear and keep on pumping.

Riding a stationary bicycle is a safe, simple means to get started. Riding indoors allows you

---

Burning It Off

Activity	Calories per hour (Gross Energy Cost)
Lying down or sleeping	80
Sitting	100
Driving an automobile	120
Standing	140
Bicycling (5½ mph)	210
Walking (2½ mph)	210
Golf	250
Bowling	270
Swimming (¼ mph)	300
Volleyball	350
Roller skating	350
Table tennis	360
Ditch digging (hand shovel)	400
Tennis	420
Water skiing	480
Skiing	600
Squash and handball	600
Cycling (13 mph)	660
Running (10 mph)	900

Source: Basic Bodywork for Fitness and Health, published by the American Medical Association.

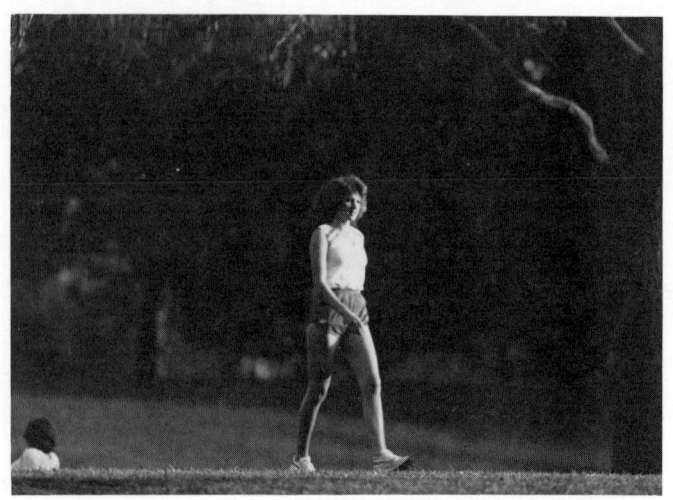

A brisk walk before dinner burns calories and creates an appetite.

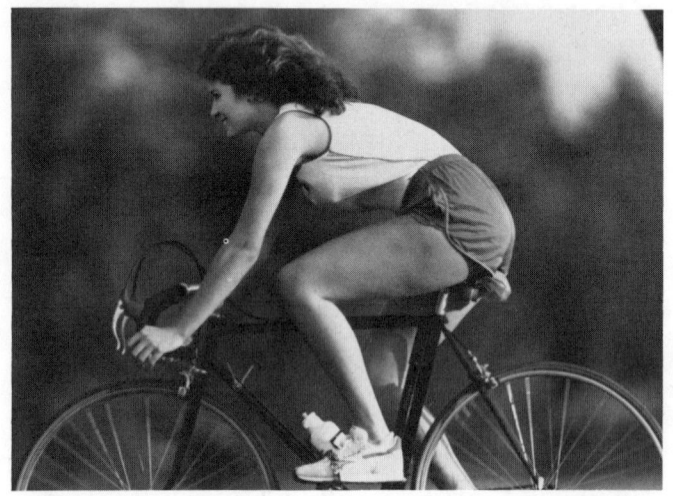

Why not ride your bicycle to work on a warm, sunny day?

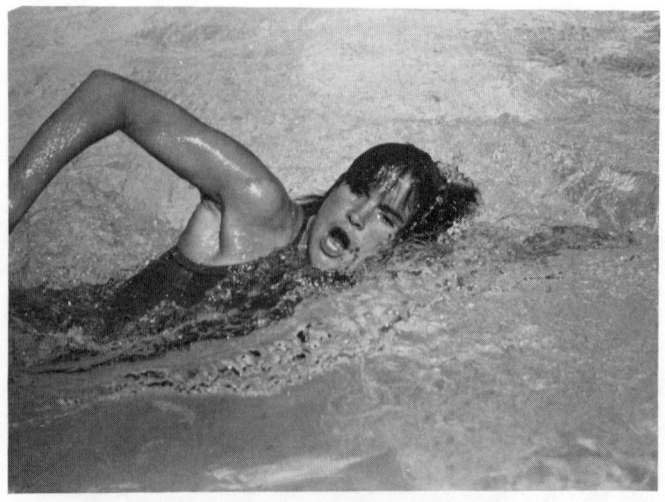

Swimming is almost an injury-free sport.

the benefits of aerobic activity without having to leave the comfort of your home or the health spa. Remember, aerobics is continuous, uninterrupted activity.

Minimum time required for aerobic benefit (both stationary and outdoor bicycling): twenty minutes.

Swimming — Not only is swimming an excellent aerobic activity, but it is also a good muscle strengthener and conditioner. And the lack of pounding or stress to the joints and muscles keeps you from sustaining any serious injuries.

Most cities and towns have indoor and outdoor public swimming pools. If you don't work, pick a time during the day and head over to the pool for a fifteen- to twenty-minute swim. Or try swimming on your lunch hour. You'll have time to shower, grab some lunch and get back to work on time.

Minimum time required for aerobic benefit: twenty minutes.

Aerobic dancing — This type of activity offers thousands of different alternatives. Whether you choose to do your workout at home to the music of your favorite record album, or with a group in a class (like Jazzercise or specialized health-club programs like Jane Fonda's Workout), aerobic dancing is just that: dance that offers the benefits of aerobics. And since you don't need to do this activity outdoors, you won't need to fret over the weather or worry about catching a cold in the rain or snow.

Surprisingly, I've heard many women say that the reason they won't consider joining an aerobic dance class is that they don't want to be seen in a leotard. If you are that self-conscious about wearing a leotard, then don't wear one! Wear some sweats or some comfortable old jeans. But don't let your vanity get in the way of what might be an enjoyable exercise program for you.

Minimum time required for aerobic benefit: fifteen minutes.

Running — About thirty million people in this country number themselves runners. Most attribute their interest to its value in gaining aerobic fitness. And rightly so: Running increases your body's capacity to use oxygen during exercise, lowers your resting pulse rate, reduces your blood pressure and increases the overall efficiency of your lungs and heart. It is one of the most efficient exercises for shedding excess pounds and toning muscles. You can also measure your aerobic improvement easily with running because times and distances are a good indication of how well you are doing.

As a runner the one pitfall you must not fall into is that of penny-pinching. Buy a good pair of shoes that offer adequate support for your body, and your body will thank you. Don't let a hungry salesperson talk you into buying a certain shoe. Try on several pair, decide which shoe fits best and is most comfortable, and buy it.

As with any other strenuous activity, it is best to start out slowly. If you have never run before, or haven't run since you were a cheerleader in high school, don't expect to be able to fly blissfully around the block. Your body needs time to ease into what it's doing. And remember to do your warm-up exercises. Running places considerable strain on the feet, legs, hips and back, and improperly stretched muscles can get pulled.

If you can't bring yourself to appear in singlet and shorts in public, then you might try running in place. If done vigorously enough (meaning lifting those knees high off the ground), running in place can have the same benefits as outdoor running. Make sure, however, that you run on a heavily padded surface and wear supportive shoes. Running in place has just as much jarring to offer as regular running.

Minimum time required for aerobic benefit (both outdoor running and running in place): fifteen minutes.

Roller or Ice-skating — If you haven't been skating since you were a kid, drag those old skates out and head to the rink. Skating is a great family fitness sport, and if done long enough to raise your pulse rate, can be a good aerobic exercise as well. Generally, though, if

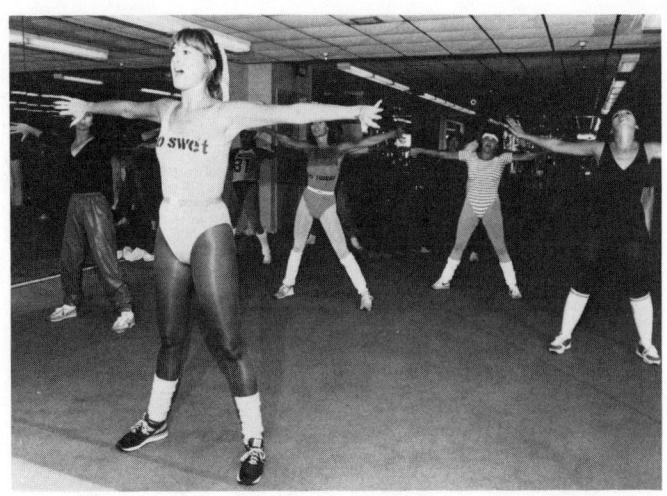

Dance aerobics is the woman's answer to enjoyable fitness.

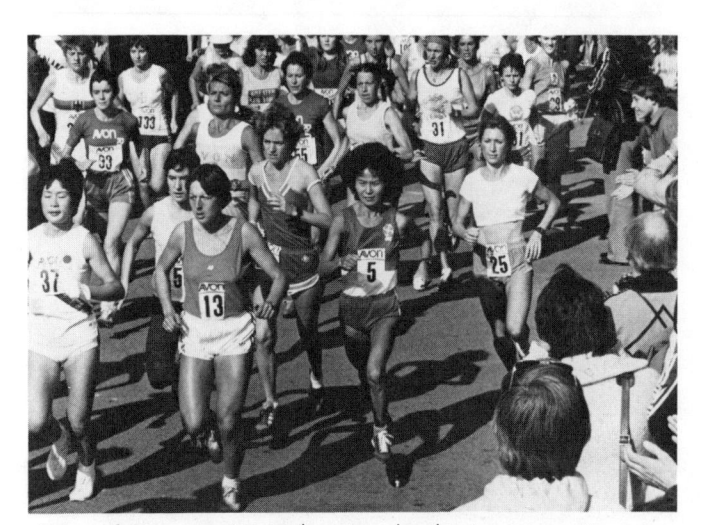

Avon, the cosmetics maker, is a leader in women's running.

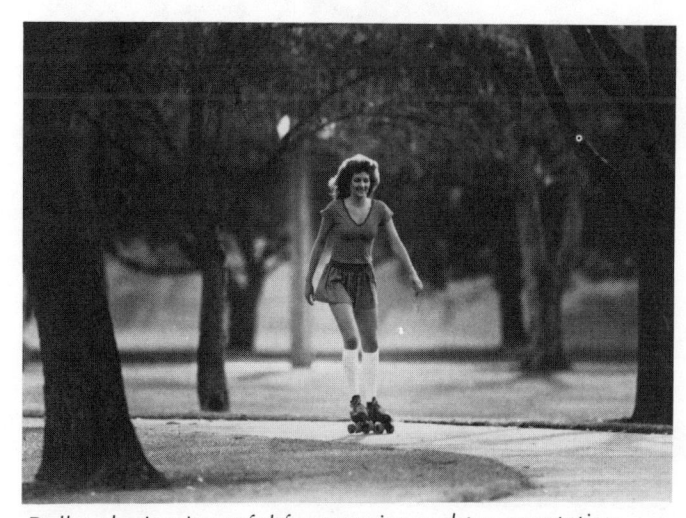

Roller skating is useful for exercise and transportation.

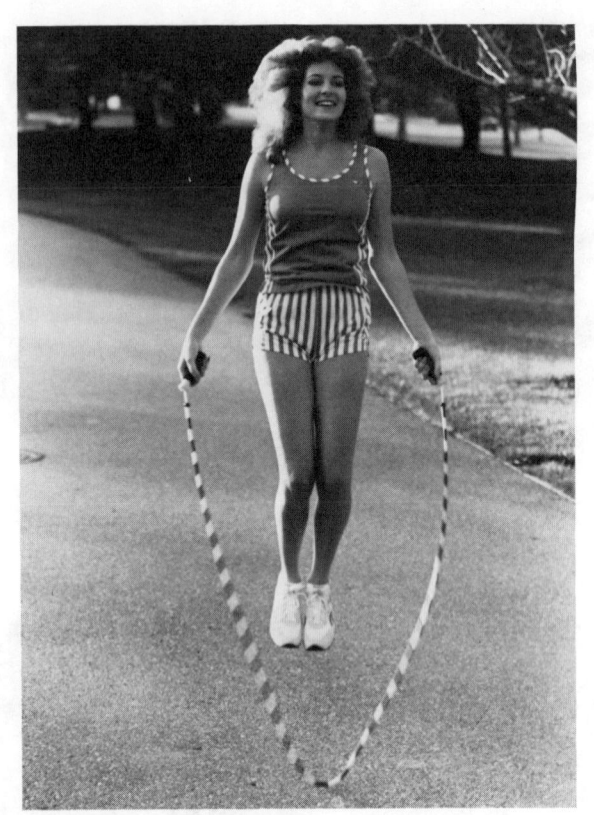

Jumping rope shapes up the leg muscles.

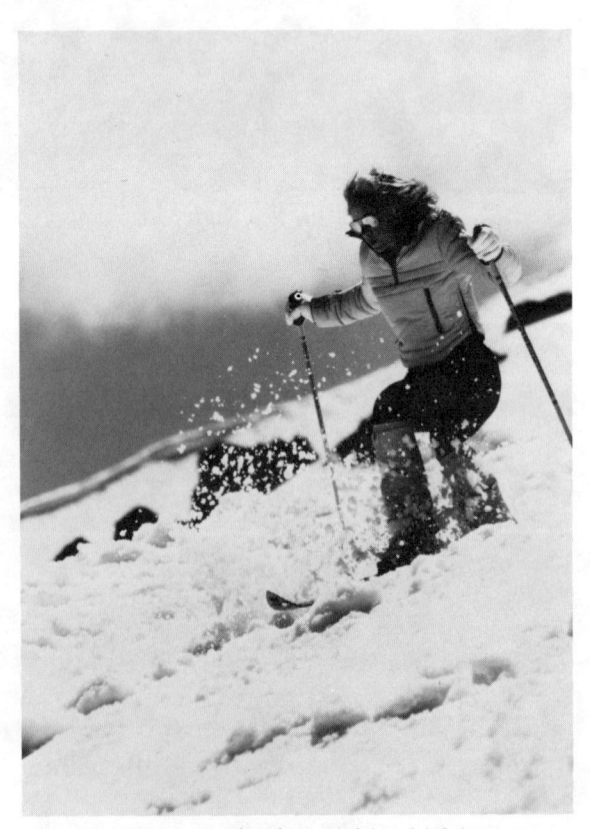

A ski vacation can be fun and healthful.

skating is your favorite activity, you should supplement it with an additional aerobic activity, such as running or aerobic dance, because we usually tend not to skate hard enough to gain aerobic benefits.

Remember your warmups once again; injuries occur for neglect of this important precaution. And always take care to wear knee pads and a helmet if you are considering taking up the sport. Spills can and do occur, too.

Minimum time required for aerobic benefit: twenty minutes.

Jumping Rope — It sounds easy, but this exercise is a lot tougher than it looks. That's one reason why it's such a good aerobic exercise. But watch out — this is a bone-jarring activity, and really shouldn't be done regularly without supplemental stretching and conditioning exercises. Make sure that when you jump, you do so on a padded surface, and wear your gym shoes so as to reduce the stress on your joints.

Both ends of the jump rope should extend to your armpits when you stand on it with both feet. If you are going to be traveling or are in a confined space, a jump rope is a nice fitness item to carry along with you. It doesn't require much room, just a lot of activity on your part.

Minimum time required for aerobic benefit: twelve minutes.

Other recreational exercises — There are many other sports that you may enjoy, such as a game of racquetball, tennis or volleyball. It is best to vary your workout to include a number of different sports and thus work different muscles, but one of your main concerns should be that of getting the all-important aerobic workout.

THE COOLDOWN

After your aerobic workout, you will notice that your heart is beating furiously and your lungs are working far more than the normal rate to bring air into the circulatory system. This is because the aerobic exercise, as mentioned before, increases your muscles' need for oxygen. Even after you have stopped your aerobic activity, however, that need for extra oxygen continues for several minutes, and this is where your cooldown becomes important. By gradually backing off on the intensity of your workout, you will not shock your system. Your muscles will be rid of built up lactic acid more quickly by cooling down and it will help reduce the chance of stiffness.

This cooldown should not be strenuous. After a fifteen-minute run, spend three to five more minutes just walking and moving your arms about to help your system get rid of lactic acid. It would feel wonderful to sit down and rest, but don't. The longer your workout, the longer should be your cooldown.

After a vigorous workout, it is also beneficial to stretch for a few minutes to keep the muscles limber. Your stretching session, however, should not be construed as your cooldown: They are separate parts of your workout and perform different functions. Do your cooldown first, to make sure that the muscles receive that added oxygen they need to get rid of lactic acid, and then do your final stretches before you take your shower.

It takes a little extra time for stretching, warming up and cooling down, but the payoff in fewer injuries makes it time well spent.

ACHIEVING GOOD MUSCLE TONE

Now that you know the importance of aerobics, warming up and cooling down, there is one more item that really should be included in your bag of health goodies: a conditioning program to tone your muscles. Conditioning consists of doing exercises that improve muscle tone by working them individually. Proper conditioning will result in muscle strength (not bulk), better posture, coordination and flexibility.

Remember that although you may feel exhausted after muscle conditioning, it does not lead to cardiovascular fitness, nor is it a substitute. Conditioning, as with warmups and cooldowns, is merely part of a good exercise program. It is a key element in achieving total fitness, along with aerobics and stretching.

So what constitutes conditioning exercises? Basically, conditioning is any form of exercise that works and stretches the muscles individually. Most calisthenics, like sit-ups, push-ups, leg lifts and toe touches, can be done for a conditioning workout. You can do it after your aerobic workout, using it as a cooldown, or in a workout separate from your aerobic exercise.

Another good method of conditioning your muscles is through weight training. I'll briefly talk about weight training here.

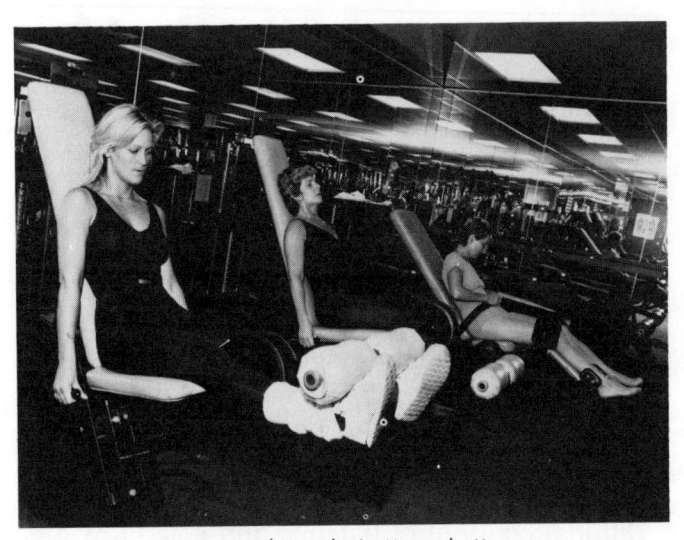

These women are working their "quads."

WEIGHT TRAINING IS FEMININE!

Many women are still under the impression that weight training is for men exclusively, and that to be seen lifting weights is the ultimate in embarrassment. Up until a few years ago that was true, but not any more!

Now is the time to dispel one myth here and now: Weight training will not make you look more masculine. Muscle overdevelopment, the effect sought after by male bodybuilders (and now some female bodybuilders) is largely controlled by the male hormone testosterone, which is not present in sufficient quantities in most women to produce bulky, ripply muscles. And those female bodybuilders that do achieve a somewhat overdeveloped musculature do so only through long hours spent lifting lots of weights. Most women, however, do not spend all of their free time in the gym; thus, they will not develop bulk.

The benefits of lifting weights, on the other hand, are endless. If you are still unsure about what lifting weights might do to your body, take a trip to your local health spa and examine the women who regularly work out with weights. You will no doubt be surprised, because they are not bulky and macho-looking, but firm, lean and usually nicely figured. Weight training is a superior conditioning method because you can firm and tone parts of your body that you can't possibly reach through doing just sit-ups and push-ups.

Take advantage of the benefits of weight training. How about a health club? Many clubs offer a separate weight room exclusively for women, if you are shy about pumping iron with the guys. The staffs of most clubs encourage women to take part in a weight training program, and will offer guidance.

At a reputable health club, you will normally find weight machines — Universal or Nautilus for example — and free weights. Both the Universal and the Nautilus equipment (among others) have the feature of more control over weight resistance. Free weights require the additional element of balance and can allow a greater range of motion compared to machines. Some people prefer combining free weights with machines during a workout. Others stick to the traditional free weights.

As you experiment with your weight training program, you will no doubt discover what is best for you. But before you begin a weight training program, ask for help. Never enter a weight room and begin using equipment that you are unfamilar with; you're asking for a big fat weight to fall on your big toe, or perhaps worse.

Once you know how to use the machines (which at first can be a little intimidating), you will enjoy working out with them. There is something to the notion that weight training builds self-confidence as it firms muscles. And if you do decide to work out in a coed facility, most often you will find that the guys not only accept you, but are willing to help you with your program. Don't be shy!

The Basic Weight Training Workout for Women

Obviously, workouts vary from woman to woman, but the following is a program using basic exercises that are applicable to everybody. Of course, before you try any of these exercises on one of the machines, ask for help, and make sure you are completely familiar with it before starting. And if you have a specific injury or sore muscle, let your instructor know, so that he can determine what exercises to avoid in your program.

It is important to warm up before beginning a workout. Weight training, as with any other exercise routine, stresses the muscles, and a good warmup of easy stretches — about five or ten minutes of your time — will get you limber for your workout.

Hip Push

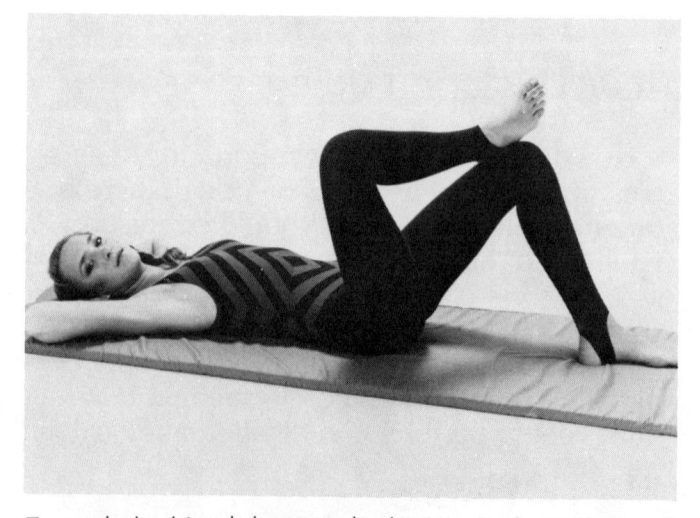

To work the hip abductors, do the Hip Push. With the crossed leg, push down on the bent leg.

Exercise 41

Fire Hydrant

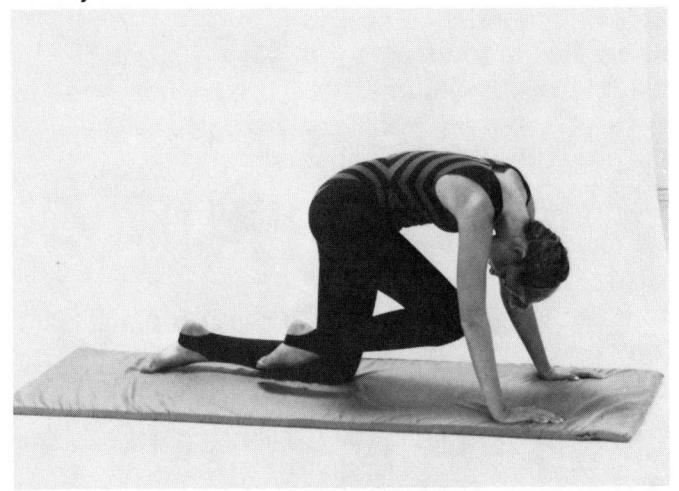

a. In Fire Hydrant, begin on all fours.

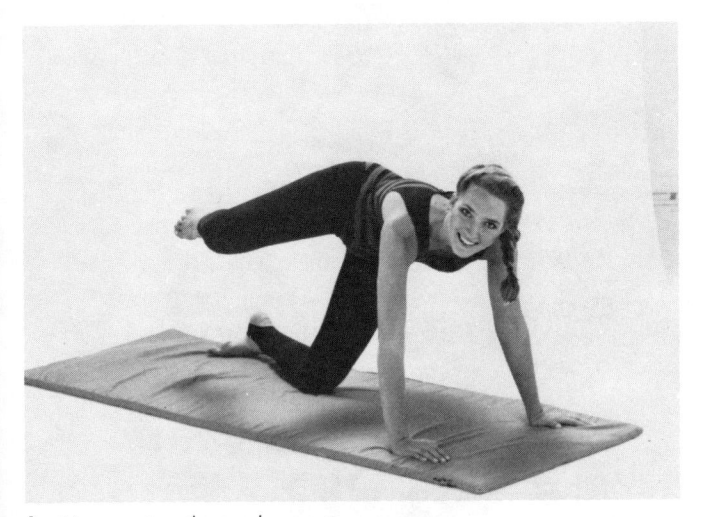

b. Now extend one leg out.

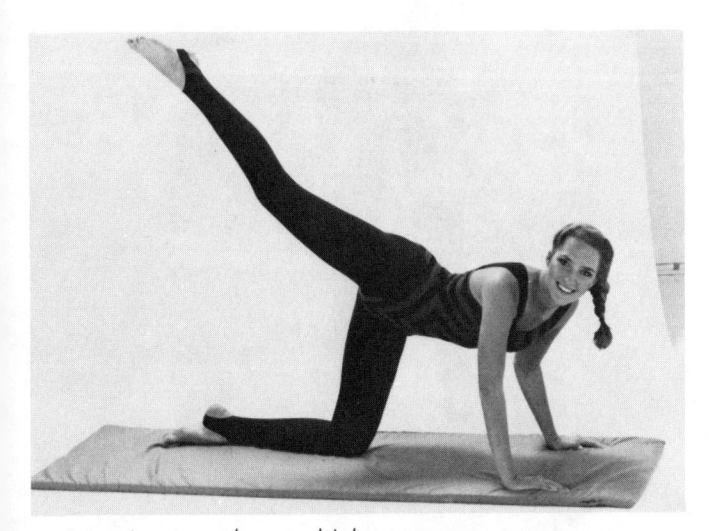

c. Bring it out and up as high as you can.

Toe Raises

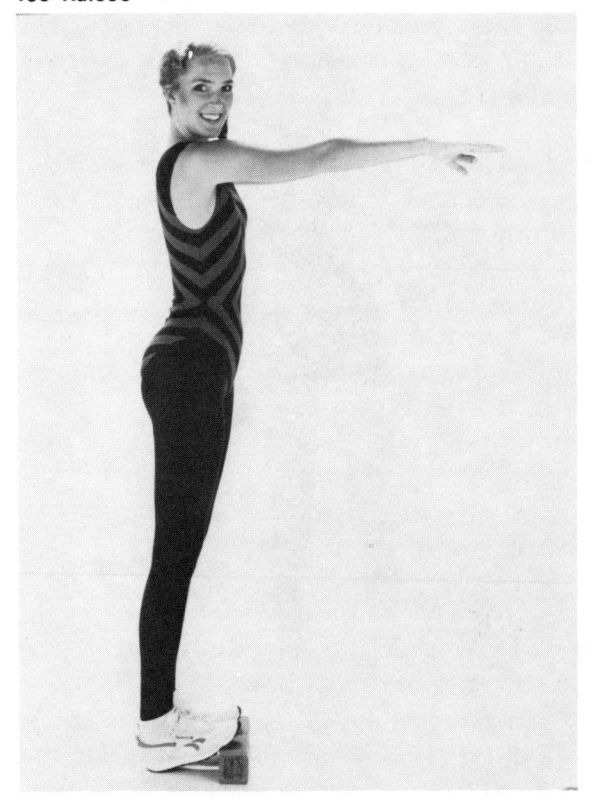

a. Toe Raises can be done on the edge of a step or block of wood.

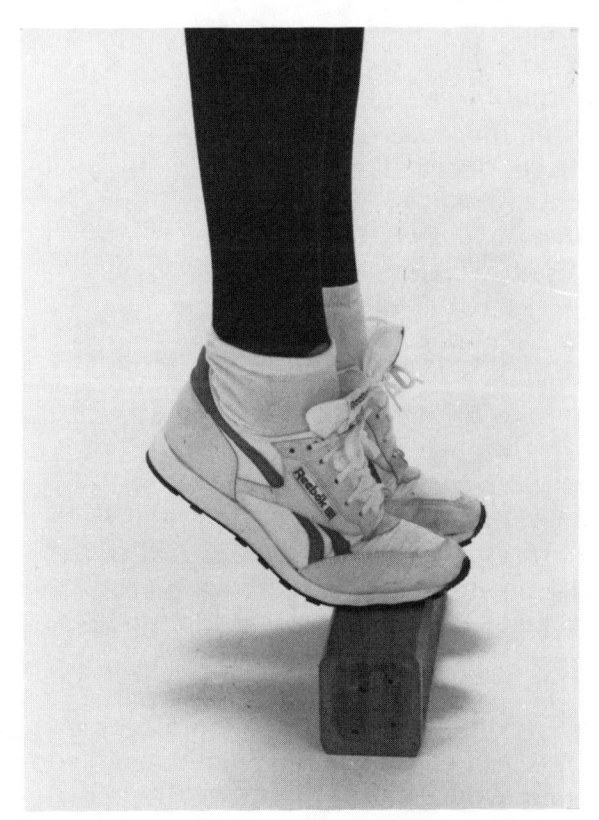

b. Raise yourself up on your toes. Repeat 10 times.

42 FIGURE MAINTENANCE

Oblique Abdominal Stretch

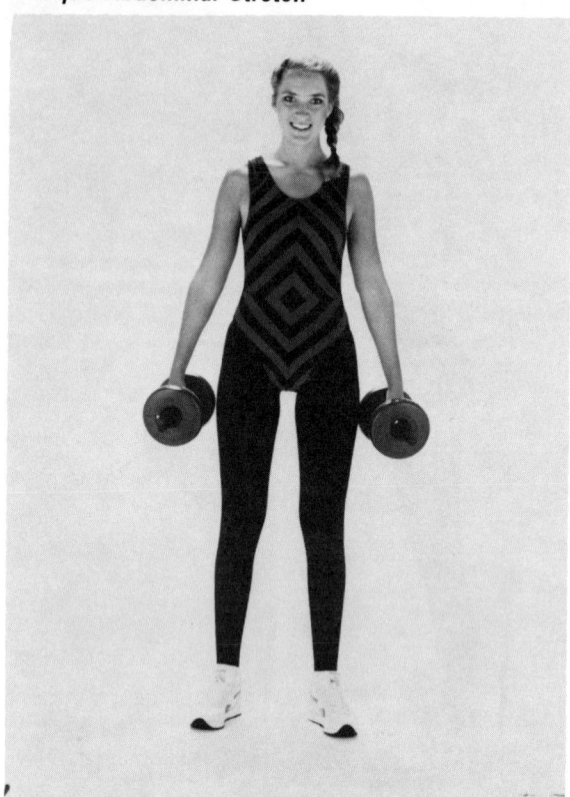

a. The oblique abdominal muscles are used here. Hold dumbbells in each hand.

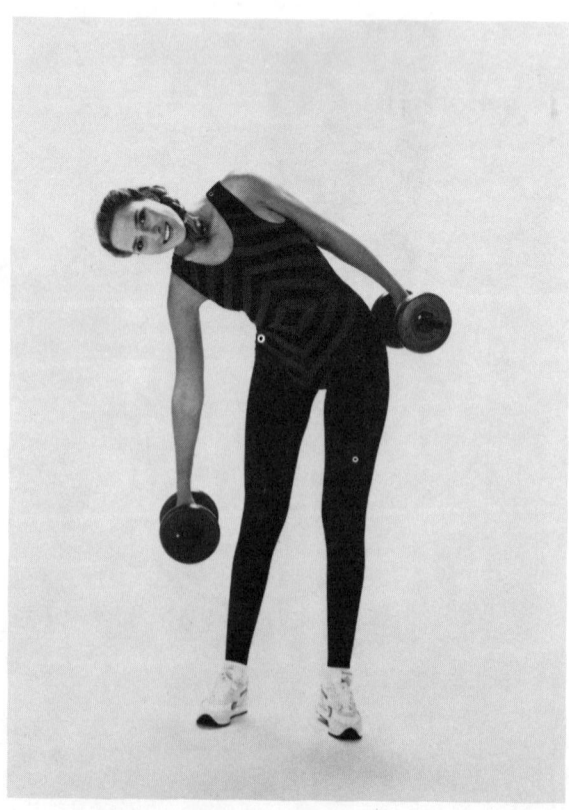

b. Now relax your arm and you will stretch the opposite side.

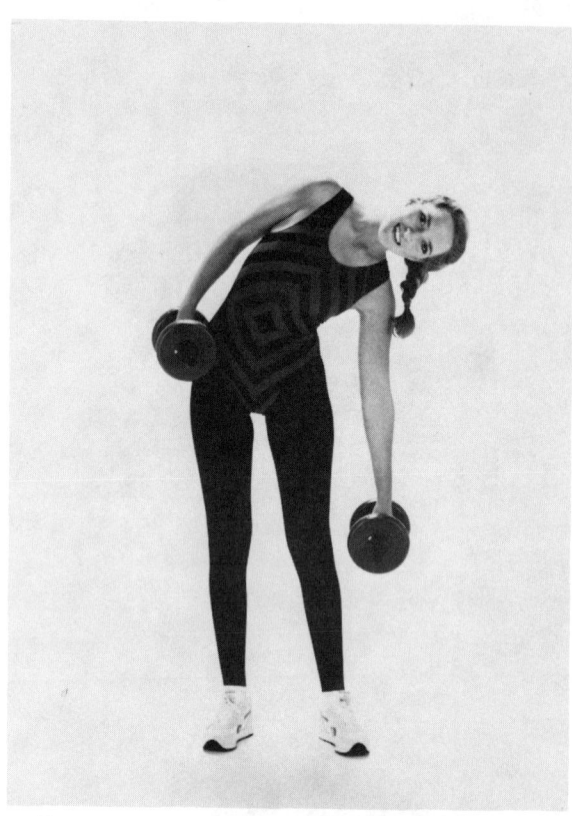

c. Return to your original position and stretch the other side.

Arm Elevators

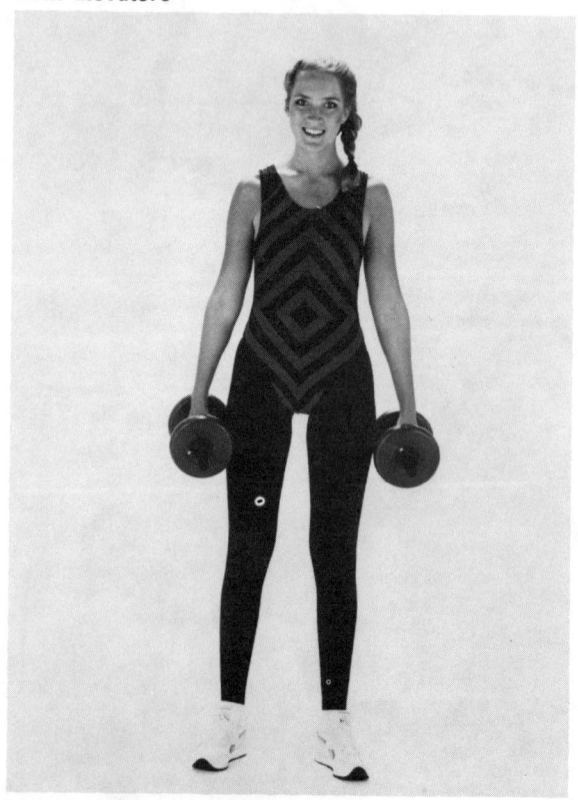

a. Arm Elevators work the deltoid muscles in the shoulder.

Exercise 43

Wing Lifts

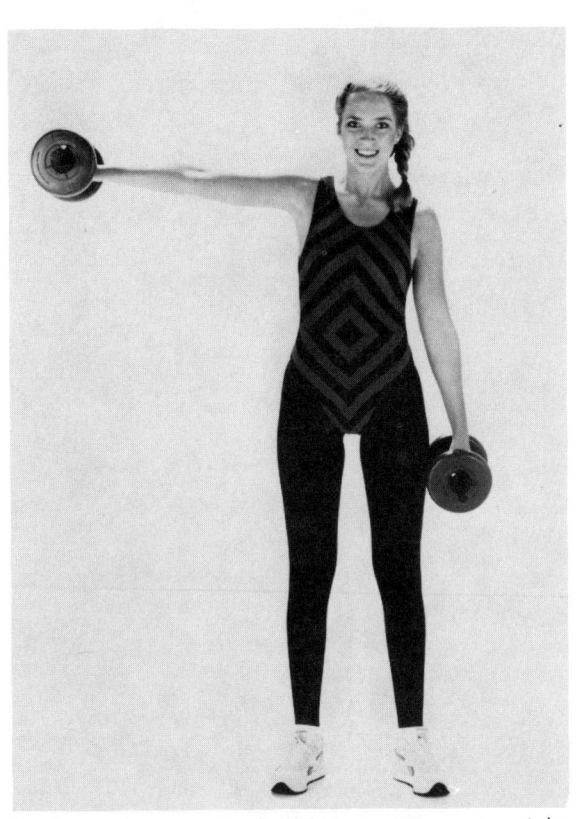

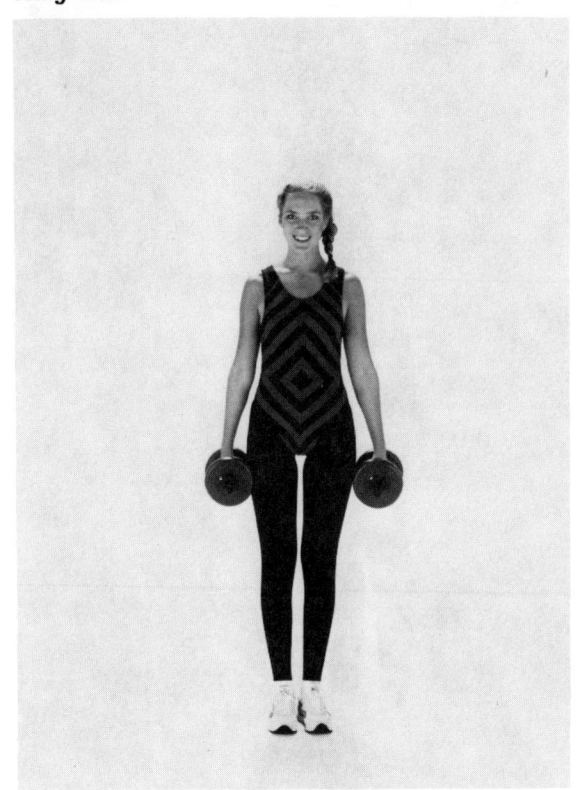

b. Begin the exercise by lifting one arm at a right angle to your side.

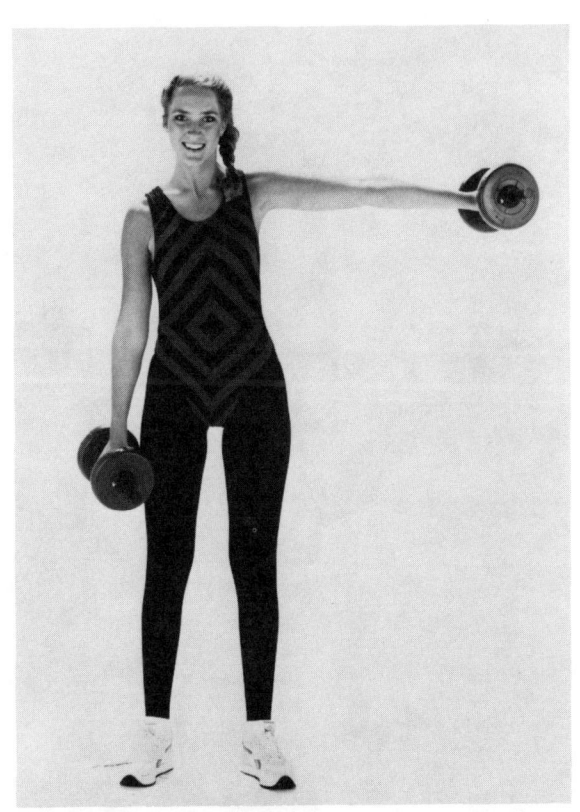

a. Wing Lifts are similar to Arm Elevators.

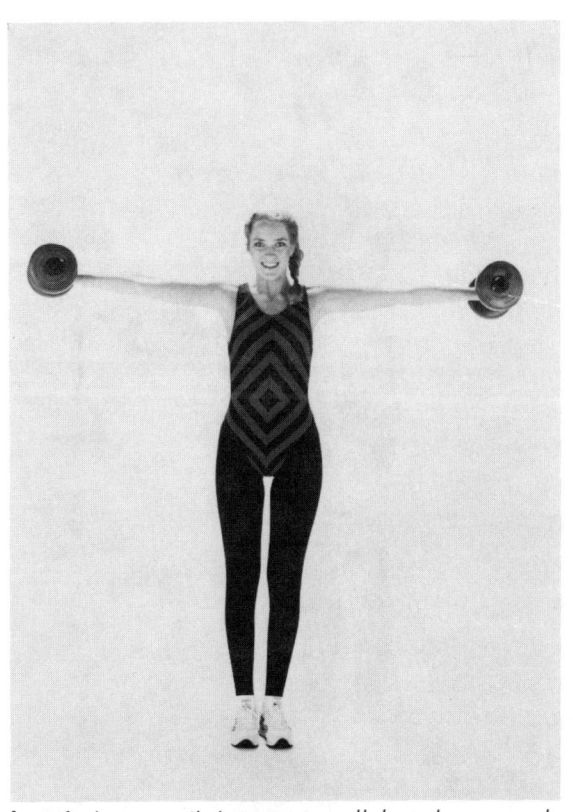

c. Return the dumbbell and work the other arm.

b. Lift them until they are parallel to the ground.

Dumbbell Curls

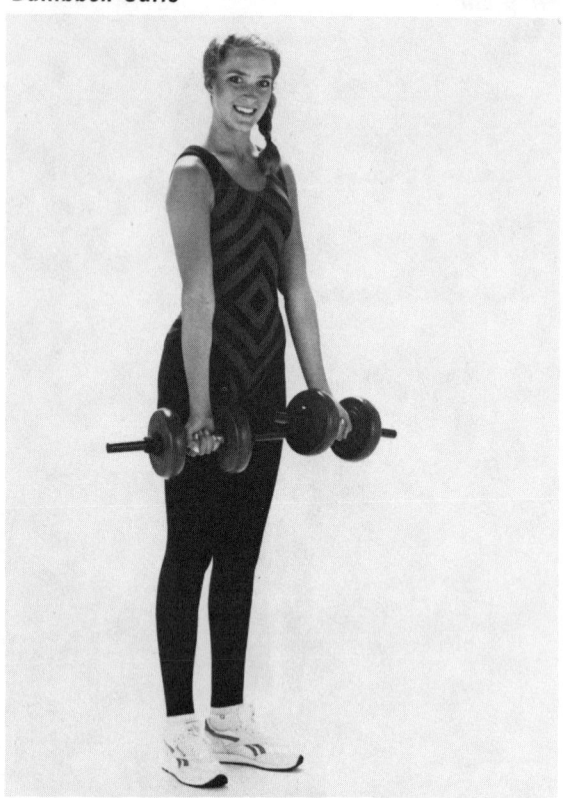

a. *Dumbbell Curls work the biceps.*

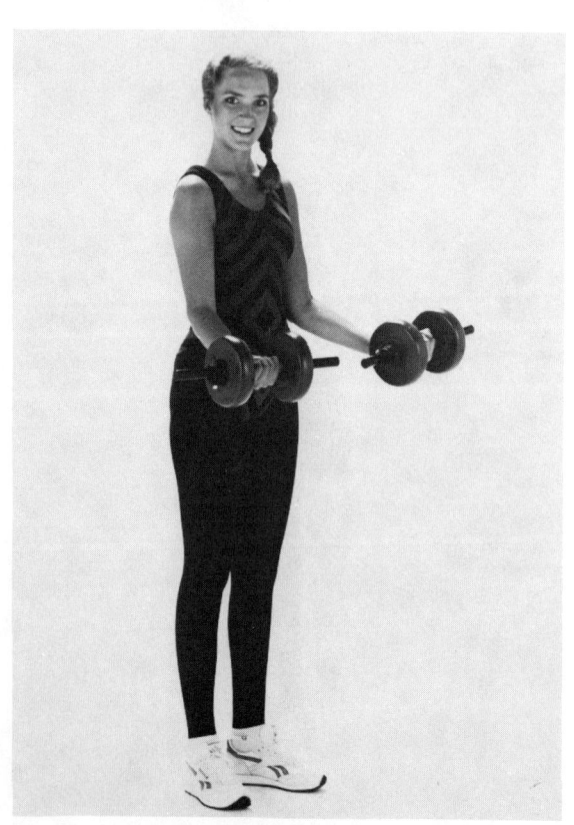

b. *Lift the dumbbells without arching your back.*

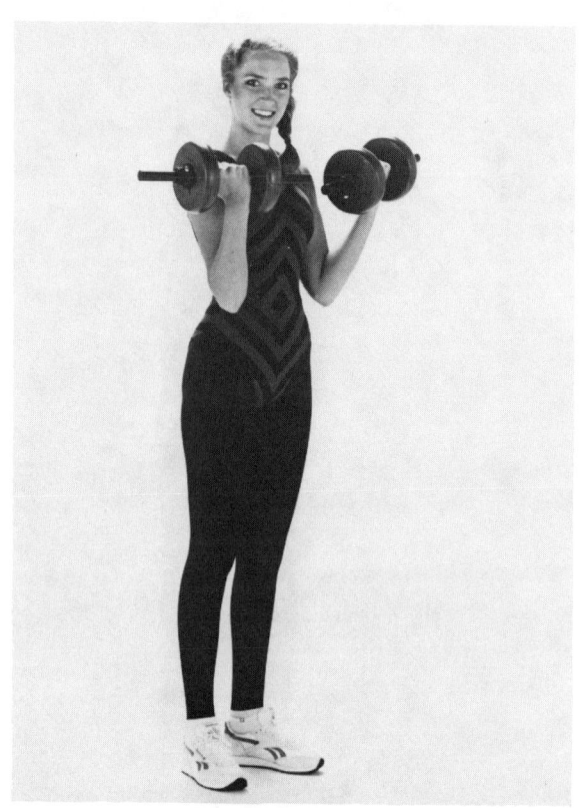

c. *Bring the dumbbells all the way up to your chin.*

Bench Press

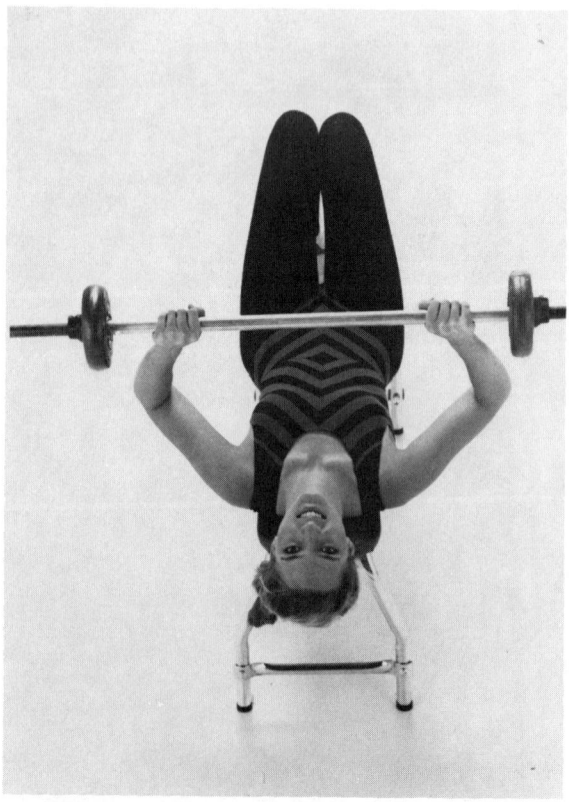

a. *To do the Bench Press using a barbell, begin with bar on chest.*

Exercise 45

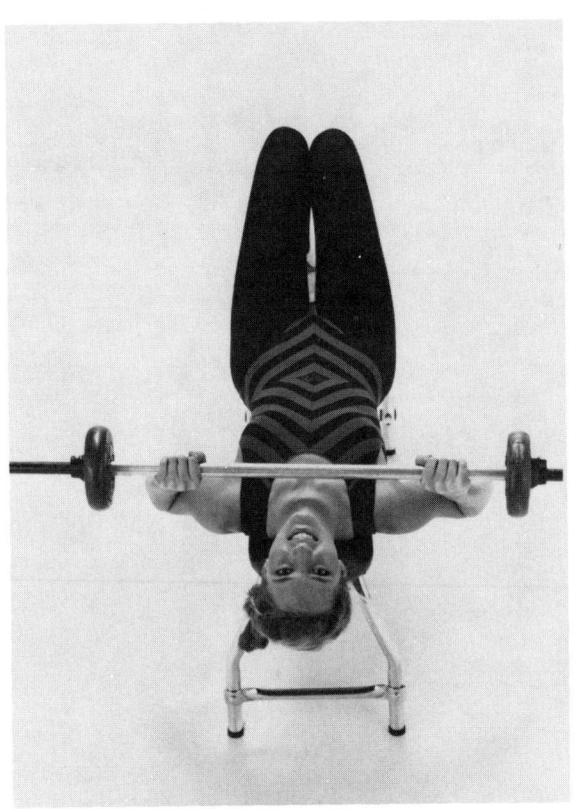

b. Have someone near you if you use a heavy weight.

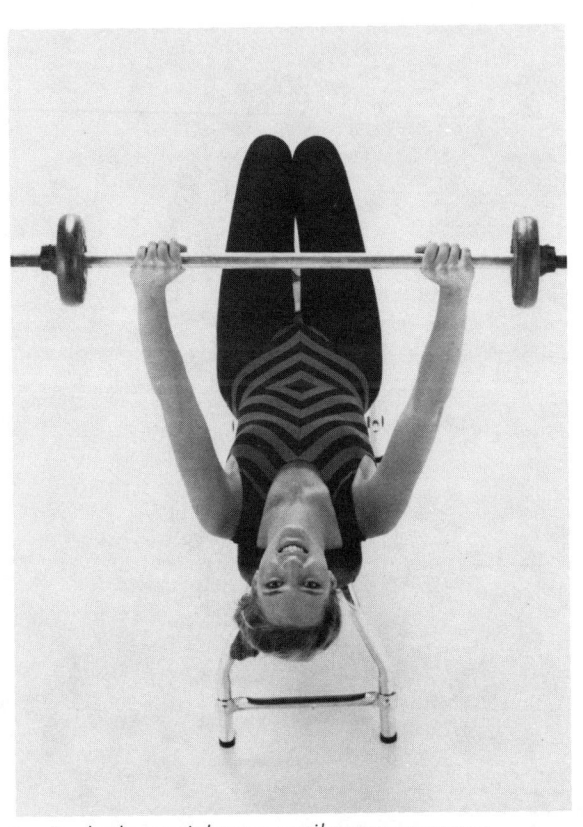

c. Push the weight up until your arms are straight. Repeat.

Back Flies

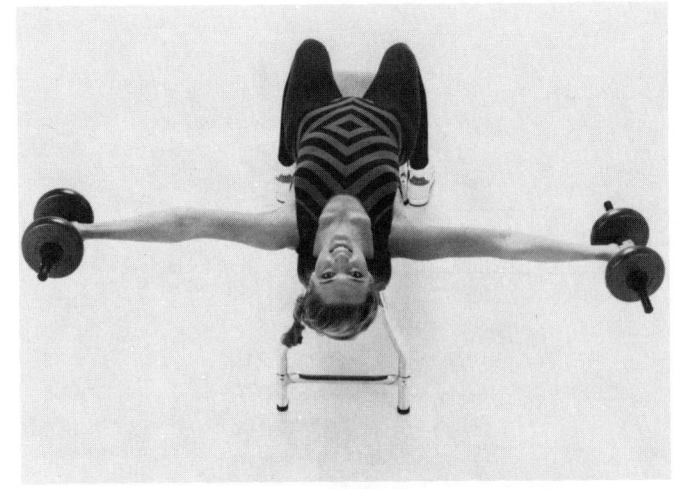

a. Back Flies are done using a bench and dumbbells.

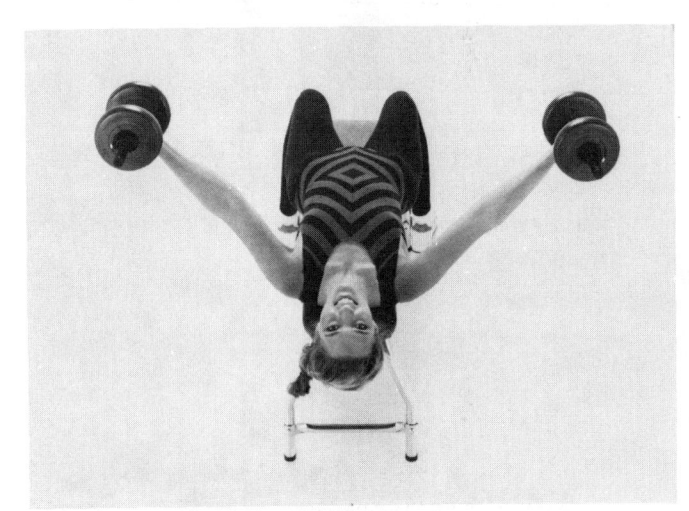

b. Bring the dumbbells simultaneously up over your head.

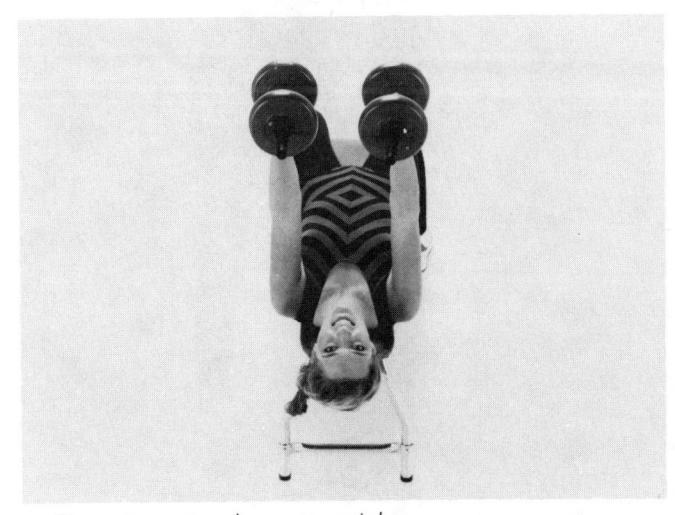

c. Do not use too heavy a weight.

Upright Rows

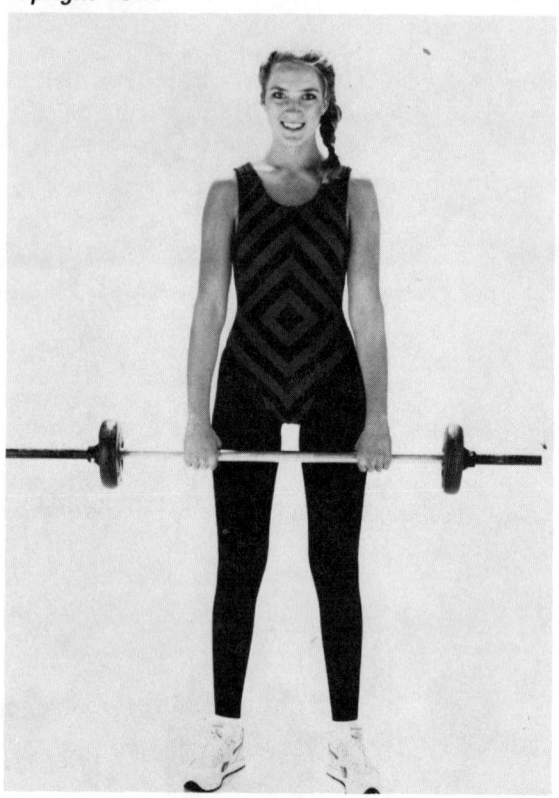

a. Begin Upright Rows with hands close together on barbell.

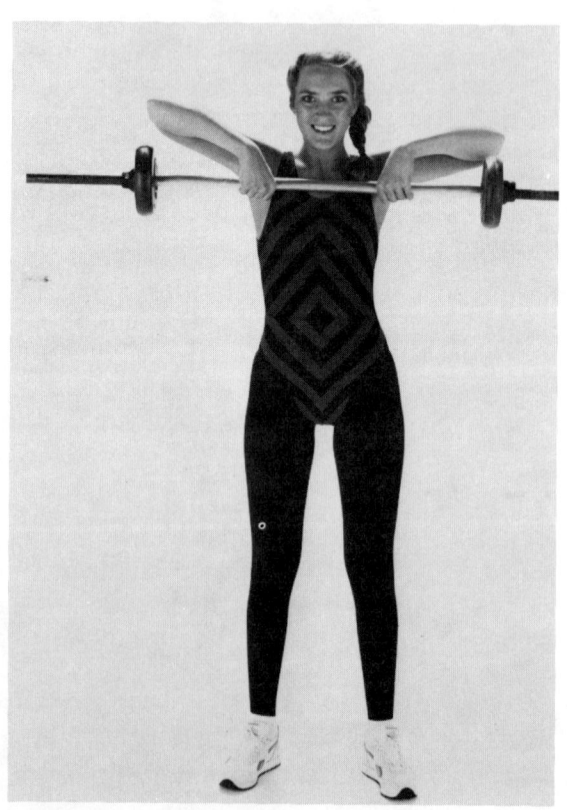

b. Lift bar slowly to chin.

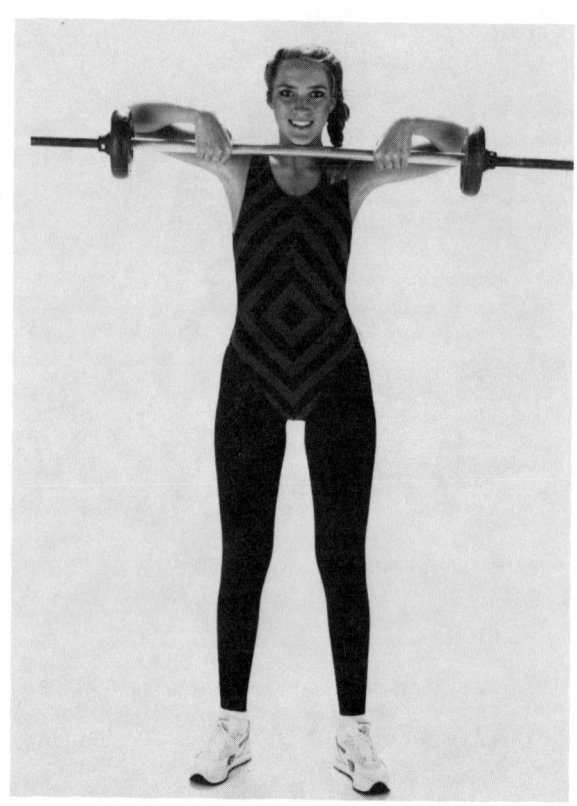

c. Upright Rows work the arms and back.

Front Raise

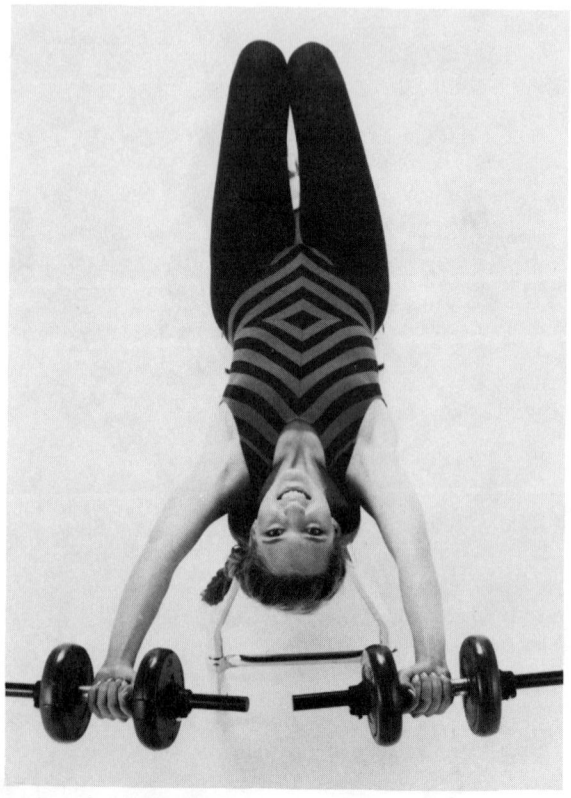

a. Do the Front Raise on your back on a bench.

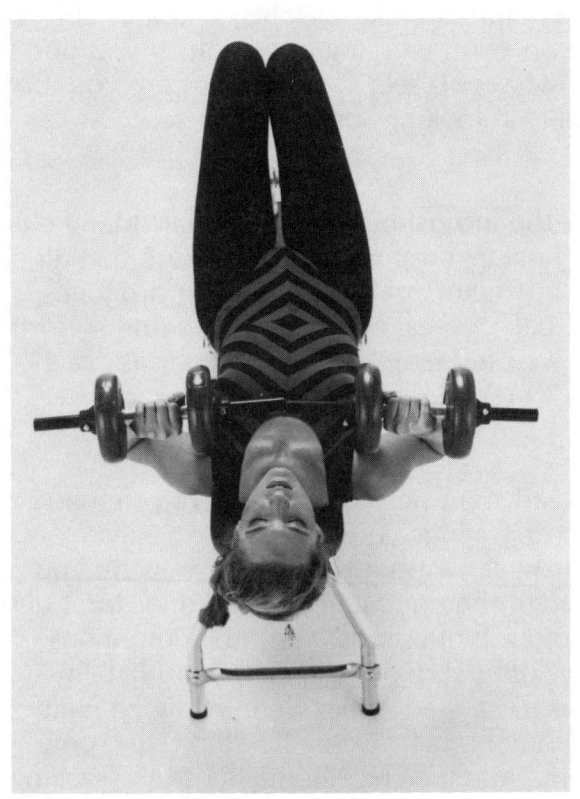

b. *Lift the dumbbells straight over your head.*

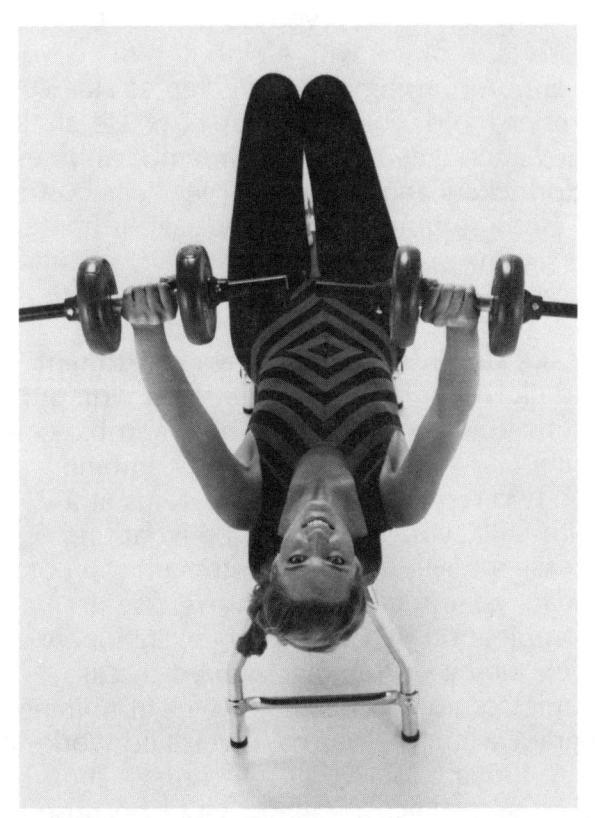

c. *Return slowly to the floor, back over your head.*

WHAT IS A GOOD HEALTH CLUB?

Now that you have learned all about the benefits of exercise, where do you do it? Many women prefer to exercise in the privacy of their homes, by themselves or with a few friends. Still others like the charged atmosphere and camaraderie that go along with working out at a health club.

Health clubs have become big business within the last few years, mainly because fitness and health has become a number one priority with people lately. But before you decide to invest in an expensive health club membership, you should be aware of what you are getting into. Health clubs range from luxurious homes-away-from-home to poorly equipped facilities that are downright unhealthy to be in. You want to make the most of your investment, so here are a few pointers to remember when considering membership in a health spa:

Weigh the alternatives. This is perhaps the most important consideration to keep in mind. First, are you going to be able to devote the time and energy it takes to make your health club investment pay off? Many women I know have forked over oodles of dollars to join an expensive club, for one reason or another, and then hem and haw and make excuses for why they can't go work out. Be sure that you are dedicated to your fitness goals; don't spend money on something that you won't benefit from.

If you don't think that you will have the time to make that investment pay off, perhaps it would be wise to consider something else. Aerobics classes, jogging clinics and other community recreational activities are generally less expensive and offer you options. The same goes for community colleges.

Be a good shopper. Don't be taken in by the first health club you visit because of its hard sell. When your car needs a diagnostic tuneup, don't you usually ask around and do some checking into several places before deciding on where you will have the work done? Be as discriminating with your body machine. Visit several health clubs in your area, ask your friends which ones they prefer, and for heaven's sake, don't be afraid to ask the club manager lots of questions. Too many people jump into a health club membership without finding out what the club has to offer. Joining a health club, like buying a car, requires a big monetary commitment on your part. It's up to you to make sure you get the most for your money.

What are your needs? What are you looking for? Consider the types of activities you are interested in pursuing. Are you a swimmer? Then you might want to find a club that has a good swimming pool. Do you like to run? Consider a club that is situated in a nice area, so that you

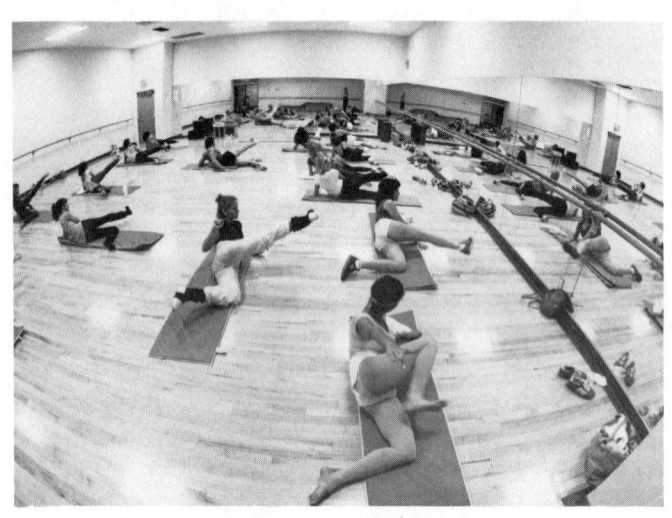

Jane Fonda's health club patrons work up a sweat.

can go out for a run after lifting weights or before playing racquetball. Be sure the club offers the kind of activities that you will be willing to spend time doing.

Do they care about you? Make sure the staff is friendly and courteous, and willing to help you establish a good program for yourself. You don't want to spend time in a place that you don't feel comfortable, and you shouldn't feel like you are imposing on the staff if you ask them for help.

Is it a nice place? Take a good look around. What are the facilities like? Are the locker rooms and shower areas clean and well equipped? Is the whirlpool cleaned regularly? Is the equipment, like weights, stationary bicycles, etc., in good working condition? If you don't like what you see, then chances are you are better off looking somewhere else.

Is the atmosphere professional? Many clubs are not staffed properly. Make sure that all of the instructors of weight training programs, racquetball classes, aerobics classes and so forth are well trained. Ask the manager about the staff's credentials.

Read the fine print. Before you sign a contract that binds you into paying a huge sum for your health club membership, be sure you read through the contract carefully, and don't hesitate to ask questions about the conditions in that contract. Does the club carry liability insurance in case of an accident involving faulty equipment, etc.? Does the club offer some type of trial membership? Sometimes by checking the club out on a trial membership basis, you can find out a lot about it before you make your down payment. Are there branches of the club in other cities? If you do a lot of moving, it is wise to hook up with a club that offers you the option of using clubs in different cities. Are membership discounts available? Is use of all facilities guaranteed with your membership fee, or do lockers and some other facilities cost extra? Get a sample contract and take it home before signing.

Make sure it's a good fitness investment. A good club should offer a diversified workout that includes the benefits of both aerobic conditioning and strength training. By combining these two types of exercise programs at a health club, you will reduce body fat and increase your flexibility and strength — your ultimate goal in taking up an exercise program. A combination of aerobic dance, stationary bicycle riding or running, with yoga, calisthenics or a good resistance weight training program will give you that diversified workout you're looking for. Don't sell yourself short because the facilities are attractive or because the instructors are good-looking. Make sure a well-rounded program is provided, so that you can meet all of your fitness goals.

By no means are we discouraging you from joining a health club. Health clubs offer the fitness-minded woman a way to get out and meet people, work out and have fun all at the same time. Just be sure you use good judgment in choosing your club.

MAKING YOUR EXERCISE PROGRAM A PART OF YOU

You've heard all about the importance of good exercise; finding out about the benefits of getting out and moving around is only part of the plan, though. The next step is completely up to you: making that exercise a part of your lifestyle. It isn't always easy. All of those excuses seem to be ever-so-important when it comes time to don those sweats or shorts and work out. But making a commitment to a fitness lifestyle means making a commitment to your body and your health, which can only be strengthened through exercise.

You'll find that once you get into the swing of an exercise program, you'll enjoy that time almost more than any other part of your day. You'll be so surprised at the marked changes in your figure and your mental attitude that any amount of discomfort during exercise will be well worth the effort.

And do chart your progress. You need an ego boost every now and then, and one of the best ways to do that is to pay attention to all the wonderful things that happen to your body when you are active. Take the time to record all your measurements before you embark on your program. And keep track of them as you begin to slim down. This will be a great incentive for you to continue with your program.

Tailor your program to your needs and interests. If you don't feel comfortable doing a certain activity, leave it out of your exercise repertoire. And try varying your activities every once in a while. The most common complaint from people who begin exercising is that it's boring. Whether it's boring or not is entirely up to you. You've got a lot of choices, so there must be an activity that suits you best. If you tried running and did not like it, don't give up exercise altogether. Move on to the next activity — perhaps bicycling or aerobic dance, but don't write off exercise on the basis of one bad experience. That's selling yourself short.

Do something nice for your body for a change. Through exercise, your body can and will look as it was meant to be: sleek, strong and beautiful.

3 STAYING HEALTHY

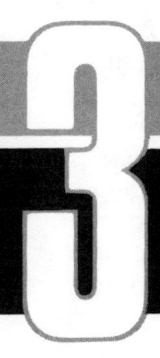

IN THE BREAKDOWN LANE

As every competitive athlete will surely attest, a body cannot run perfectly forever. At some point in time, for one reason or another, it says "Enough is enough," and slows down a little bit. It gets tired and cranky, kind of like an old car that just doesn't have enough "oomph" to get itself moving.

At this point, you should be very careful with what you ask of your tired old body. If you are very active and exercise frequently, this is crucial. Your body is highly susceptible to injury in its fatigued state. Injuries occur most often to active people when their bodies are at a low point, perhaps brought about by too much exercise, from a recent illness or from stress and strain.

As an active person who is concerned about her body, you should make every effort to become aware of its moods and whims. Plain and simple: When you work your body too hard, when you train too long or too fast, when you overexert and overuse your body's storehouse of energy, you are going to get hurt.

But don't think that you have no recourse but to sit back and let this happen. Learn to read your body's signals and you can avoid injury. Your body gives you every chance (usually) to figure out what is going on and to change your plan of action before something drastic happens, like a muscle pull, a sprain or a nagging, lingering illness.

Many people will tell you that ignoring these warning signals will cause them to disappear and that, in fact, you will return to normal. I can't rule out that possibility, but more often than not, when you ignore your body signals the result is something bad. And the more you ignore your body's needs, the more the chances of an injury occurring. The cumulative effect of stress and overuse on the body can even lead to serious injuries, and who needs that?

So what are some of these body signals? In general terms, pay attention to your body functions as a whole. Ask yourself what changes are going on inside of you.

• Are your exercise sessions or workouts becoming increasingly difficult to handle? Are you finding that you cannot train as much today as you did last week?

• Are you losing an inordinate amount of weight? (Don't laugh — although this is our objective when we begin an exercise program, excessive weight loss can signal trouble.)

• Are you experiencing difficulty in falling asleep, or sleeping fitfully?

• Are you experiencing considerable pain during your workouts? Although proper exercise does involve the application of stress to our bodies, there is a practical limit. Let pain be your limiting factor. Too much pain means it's time to back off.

- Are you feeling rundown and tired, even after your workout? Your standard workout should leave you feeling invigorated and full of energy. When fatigue sets in even before a workout, your body is probably on the downslide and begging for rest.

- Are your eating habits changing drastically? You should know how much you eat. If you are eating more or less than normal, that's an indication of a definite problem.

- And how about your nerves? Have you been having trouble relaxing lately; are you irritable with friends, loved ones or workmates; does life in general seem like "a bummer"? When your "psychological resilience" is at a low point, your body will feel the effects also, and this is perfect time to get slapped with that injury.

It's all a matter of troubleshooting. No one knows what's going on inside your body except you, and if you don't pay attention, who will? You know when your body is feeling out of sorts, and sometimes you can prevent an injury by doing a little of this troubleshooting. Now, that doesn't mean that just because you listen to your body signs that you will always be able to avoid an injury; some injuries cannot be helped. But a surprising majority of athletic injuries are incurred because the body is just not feeling up to par.

There is a tendency, too, for athletically-inclined women to mask those signs of body stress and overuse by working themselves even harder, under the premise that if they toughen themselves sufficiently, they will make their bodies immune to injury and illness. Not true. Ask any competitive athlete. Most probably, they will tell you that they tried that approach, and that after they pulled muscles in their legs and backs, they decided to give that old body what it was demanding — rest!

RESTING TIRED OLD BONES

Resting does not mean crawling into bed and staying there for several days. It just means giving the body a chance to catch up with you.

RECOVERY TIMES

1. Distance of Race	2. Minimum Recovery Period	3. Minimum Time Recommended Until Next Race
2 miles	24 hours	3 days
5 miles	3 days	7 days
10 miles	7 days	2 weeks
15 miles*	2 weeks	1 month
Marathon**	1 month	3 months
50 miles***	3 months	1 year

*Not more than 5 15-milers recommended per year.
**Not more than two all-out marathons per year.
***Not more than one 50-miler every two years.

If you are a runner, be careful that your are not pushing yourself too hard. This chart gives an idea of the minimum amount of time needed for rest before and after races of varying distances. Make sure you're protecting yourself against injuries!

Source: The Complete Runner (World Publications, 1974)

That may mean taking up another less strenuous activity for a while, or it may mean laying off your workout for a couple days or a week. And you needn't feel that you are "robbing" your body by not working out. Your body needs rest at this point, not a workout. And no one really needs to subscribe to self-abuse.

If you are working out hard every day, you are inviting injury. Do one easy day and one hard day, alternating with this pattern throughout the week. Or skip a day altogether. If you have already suffered an injury, you will have to do this, if not stop altogether for a while. But if you haven't, this is a smart way to avoid that possibility. Substitute another activity. If you run five days a week, try something like weightlifting or swimming every other day. Sometimes this will give the body the break it needs without having to completely stop your activity.

Don't be stubborn with yourself. When we lock ourselves into an exercise routine, we tend to get very "dedicated" to our cause, and that dedication makes us suffer through even the most agonizing workouts. This dedication is wonderful, but don't mistake dedication for stubbornness. If you are injured, back off. There will always be another day for your

Staying Healthy 53

workout; besides, if you work out when you are injured, you could make the injury much worse. Then it will take much longer to get well. One or two days of rest — even a week — will not upset your fitness goals. In fact, rest is the key to improvement, to allow the body to rebuild itself.

As always, eat a well-balanced diet. Sometimes eating the right foods can make all the difference in the world. The same is true of eating the wrong foods. Eating too many rich, fatty foods, for example, is like pouring sludge into your car oil. It will gum up the works. The body has to work doubly hard to process this "fuel."

If you're in the middle of a workout and begin to feel exhausted — really exhausted — don't tough it out. Stop for a few minutes or, if necessary, stop altogether. You are increasing your risk of injury by continuing. You know how hard you normally work while exercising, so pace yourself. Remember, that is one of the key points of a good exercise program — it shouldn't be excruciatingly painful.

TIME FOR REPAIRS

No matter how conscientious you are, there is going to be the occasional injury. Many people get mad at themselves and become irrational when this happens. They refuse to get medical help when it is obviously called for. Although many injuries require nothing more than time and rest to heal, a visit to the doctor is a reasonable precaution.

Doctors and other members of the medical profession were once sacrosanct. You never questioned their diagnosis or treatment. Happily, that is no longer so. As with any other financial investment, you should probably shop around to assure yourself that you have found the best possible care and treatment. Most doctors are knowledgeable and respected professionals, others are quacks.

When you consider selecting a specialist to treat a specific problem, or even if it's just a general practitioner you need, ask yourself the following questions:

"Is this physician well-qualified?" There are several directories available in libraries that can be used to help you locate a qualified physician in your area, the most well-known of which is the American Medical Association's *Directory of Medical Specialists*. Through research you can find out just exactly what are a doctor's credentials. It's not snooping — it's your body that this doctor will be dealing with. Would you ask a mechanic to work on your car without first checking out his credentials?

The medical world is filled with specialists now, so ask yourself what you need. If you have a sore knee from your running, for example, then you might want to look up a sportsmedicine specialist or an orthopedic surgeon instead of a general practitioner. Specialists will have a better understanding of your injury and how to treat it than would a general practitioner or family doctor.

"Is this physician well informed?" The medical profession of today is light years more modern than the one just a decade ago. Discoveries and findings are made on a daily basis, some of them pointing to new ways of evaluating and treating disease and injury. With so much research going on in the field of medicine, it is hard to find a physician who keeps up with the times. But look for one who at least makes the attempt.

Medical literature is one of the best means by which a doctor keeps up with the rapidly changing medical world. Look to see if there are any books and, especially, medical journals in your doctor's office. *The American Journal of Medicine, New England Journal of Medicine, Annals of Internal Medicine,* and *Journal of the American Medical Association (JAMA)* are some of the major publications of the medical field. Ask for any literature that pertains to your particular problem, and see if any recent developments have been made for treating your ailment, or for its prevention. Prevention should be the cornerstone of the medical profession, not treatment of symptoms. Your doctor should know a lot about preventive medicine.

"Does this physician have a good reputation?" Nobody can tell you more about a doctor's skills and ability than another person who has patronized that physician. Just as you would ask your friends about their cars when you are looking for a new automobile, ask your friends about the particular doctor that you have been thinking about seeing. You can also ask someone you know and trust who has had a problem similar to yours to recommend a doctor. The more opinions you get the better.

"Does this physician care about my needs?" A good doctor is readily available when you need his services. Bad doctors are always out playing golf. A good doctor will seem as concerned with your medical care as you are with your problem. A bad doctor will tell you it's all in your head and that you're upsetting his game.

4 STRESS AND RELAXATION

THE FINE TUNING: FITNESS FOR THE MIND AND THE PEACE OF MIND

Mind and Body: Forever Linked

Since the Middle Ages, and probably even before that, philosophers, doctors and wise men of the day have tended to separate the functions of the mind and the body. And to this day we still cling to those separations of powers. We have physical activity — in which we use our bodies — and we have mental activity — which requires the use of our minds. For maladies of the body, we entrust ourselves to the care of physicians, and for ailments of the mind, we will ask help of a psychiatrist or psychologist.

This has been our way of thinking, but doesn't that seem to be a fragmented view of the human being? How much better would it be if we considered the person as a whole, rather than dividing her into little pieces?

Similarly, a healthy attitude toward fitness is not complete without concentrating on the needs of the mind and spirit. Fitness means being fit both in mind and in body. How can you feel the total benefits of physical fitness if you're in a "bad head space"? How can you pursue your body's health and fitness goals if don't have the right positive mental outlook to persevere for those goals?

THE STRESSES AND STRAINS OF EVERYDAY LIFE

It would be much easier if we all had good mental attitudes. Then we wouldn't have to worry about the problem of separation of mind and body. What holds us back probably more than anything else is stress. A certain amount of stress is good for us; more than that and it's all debilitating.

Stress takes many forms in our lives. Sometimes it attacks fiercely; other times it creeps up on you like a stealthy cat. Nor is stress the same for all people. For some, stress may come from the job; for others, home life may be what ties your mind and stomach in knots. It may come from the unfulfilled goal, the unexpected outcome of a particular event, or the effect that a person or several persons has on us. In short, just about everything in our world can cause stress if we let it.

What does all this have to do with physical fitness? Well, it's not enough to say that the mind undergoes stress; the body is also affected. In our fast-paced, modern society, an awareness is finally developing that mental stresses have a direct effect upon the body.

Be your own best example. Think about something that really worried you, that really had you in a frazzle. Perhaps that all-important

Holmes/Rahe Social Readjustment Ratings

Life Event	Answer		Intensity
Death of spouse	yes	no	100
Divorce	yes	no	73
Marital separation	yes	no	65
Jail term	yes	no	63
Death of close family member	yes	no	63
Personal injury or illness	yes	no	53
Marriage	yes	no	50
Fired from work	yes	no	47
Marital reconciliation	yes	no	45
Retirement	yes	no	45
Change in family member's health	yes	no	44
Pregnancy	yes	no	40
Sex difficulties	yes	no	39
Addition to family	yes	no	39
Business readjustment	yes	no	39
Change in financial status	yes	no	38
Death of close friend	yes	no	37
Change to different line of work	yes	no	36
Change in number of marital arguments	yes	no	35
Mortgage or loan over $10,000	yes	no	31
Foreclosure of mortgage or loan	yes	no	30
Change in work responsibilities	yes	no	29
Son or daughter leaving home	yes	no	29
Trouble with in-laws	yes	no	29
Outstanding personal achievement	yes	no	28
Spouse begins or stops work	yes	no	26
Change in residence	yes	no	20
Change in schools	yes	no	20
Change in recreational habits	yes	no	19
Change in church activities	yes	no	19
Change in social activities	yes	no	18
Mortgage or loan under $10,000	yes	no	17
Change in sleeping habits	yes	no	16
Change in number of family gatherings	yes	no	15
Change in eating habits	yes	no	15
Vacation	yes	no	13
Christmas season	yes	no	12
Minor violation of the law	yes	no	11

Now go back over the chart and circle the intensity point value of each yes answer, and add up the total. The higher the total, the greater the chances of your being under enough stress to make you physically ill. Holmes and Rahe found that people scoring around 150 had about one chance in three of developing a serious stress-related illness in the next two years.

job interview, an appointment in court, or the fact that you didn't meet a particular deadline. Think about how your body felt at the time. If you are like most people, that stressful situation was rooted not only in your mind, but in your body as well. You might have had pounding migraine headaches, or your stomach felt like it had been turned inside out. You could have felt tired.

The reason for your body's negative reaction to stress is what has been called the "fight or flight" syndrome, a primitive response to fear and physical danger that we humans share with every other creature on this planet. At the sign of danger (in this case, the stressful situation), your body prepares you for rapid, intense activity. Pulse rate and breathing quicken. Blood pressure elevates. Digestive processes slow down, and your circulation pumps blood away from the internal organs and concentrates it in the muscles. Muscles tense, as a result, while the blood sugar level increases to provide you with the extra fuel you need for exhausting physical activity.

The worst thing about this process is that it happens automatically, without regard for what else is going on in the body at the time. Stress is predictable; it acts in much the same way each time. What's more, this "fight or flight" response automatically wipes just about everything else from your mind when you are under stress, so that all of your thought processes are concentrated on the problem. That in turn makes that stress' effects on your body that much more focused and intense.

It is not hard to see that this situation can become damaging. As the mind is stressed repeatedly, the fight or flight response gradually begins to erode your physical equilibrium. If the stresses continue, the body begins to break down, leading to such stress-related medical problems as coronary heart disease, chronic high blood pressure, severe gastric ulcers, stroke, and so on.

The picture looks bleak, doesn't it? If this response triggers automatically, then can we stop it at all? That's a personal question, but when you are making a commitment to fitness, you are making a commitment to total fitness, not just fitness for your arms and legs. Stress is a problem that you, as a fit person, have to deal with.

Actually, one of the best answers to the question of how to reduce stress makes common sense. In the fight or flight response, your body prepares itself for heavy physical activity. So why not carry through on that? Right — go out and exercise. Participating in a vigorous aerobic activity will help you to iron out those stress-related kinks. Exercise is a natural process for bringing about relaxation.

However, most of you don't have time to throw on your running shorts and go out and pound the streets for twenty-five minutes every single time you are affected by stress. There just isn't the time, for the majority of you, to exercise out the consequences of all the stresses that play on you each day. Don't worry. Exercising four to five days a week is enough of a vent to allow the body to handle almost any level of stress. Half the battle is recognizing that stress is affecting your life and doing something about it. We can't forever eliminate stress but we can at least learn to deal with it when it comes along.

LEARNING TO RELAX

Relax — that's an easy enough word to say. Unfortunately it's much easier to say than it is to do. Our lives run at rapid-fire pace — the pressures of work, social and home atmospheres swirl about us at such a constant rate that it seems like none of us has time to think about relaxing.

But relaxing is an important part of being able to cope with the world we live in without letting the stresses around us damage the health of our minds and bodies. Life is a series of stresses, and, amazingly, without stress we would all wither up and die very quickly. Consider the bedridden elderly person: Without activity in his life, he has no reason to live. But we have to learn to strike a happy medium between a life empty of goals and letting stress kill us. Relaxation every once in a while is the key to striking that balance.

But how to relax? Good question. If relaxing were easy to explain and do, there probably wouldn't be as many stress-related diseases plaguing our society today. Each person will have her own particular likes and dislikes, and no one likes to relax in quite the same way. Where a long, invigorating hike in the mountains might be the perfect relaxing getaway for one, a day spent napping on the couch in front of the television might do the trick for another.

When you think about relaxing, what's the first thing that comes into your mind? How do you like to relax? This is probably the best way to find out what will work best for you. If you haven't thought about it lately, like many of us, then the following section will be of interest to you, and it might help you to figure out how you can make time for some productive relaxation.

MAKING TIME FOR YOURSELF

In this workaday world of ours, we hurry and scurry from one important business affair to another. We rush around, attending to the needs of everyone except ourselves. Our body and mind cry out for some loving care, but all too often we are so busy keeping up with all the little things in our lives that we neglect to listen to our own mind and its needs.

Listening to yourself is an important part of learning how to relax. Knowing that your mind and body need a rest, and that they need to be soothed every now and then, is the next step in battling stress. If you think you haven't been listening to yourself lately, see how you answer these questions:

• Are you a constant hurrier? Is there *never* enough time in a day to get everything done?
• Do you find yourself often getting hostile with your co-workers or your loved ones?
• Do you find the need to always be doing two things at one time, like reading the paper while eating, or paying bills while talking on the phone?
• Do you constantly compete with those around you, no matter what the situation?
• Do you find yourself comparing your own successes and accomplishments with those of others — a lot?
• Do you avoid getting "involved" with other people?

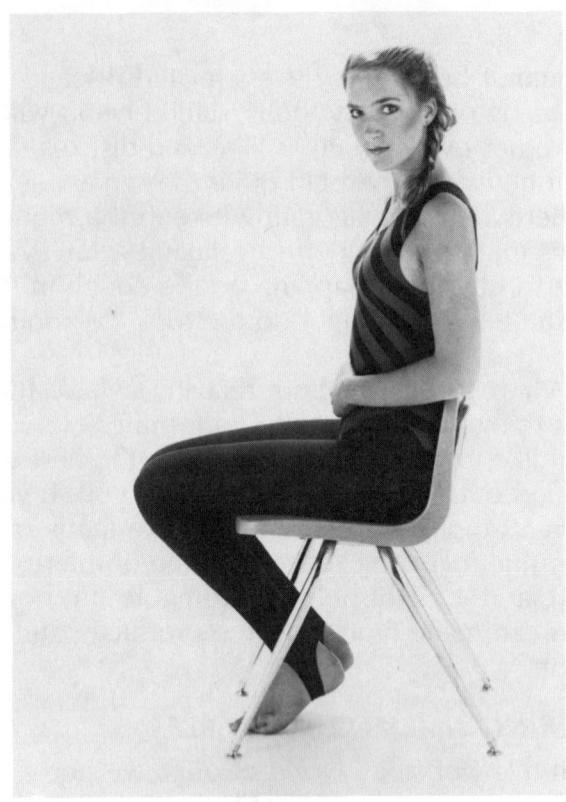

Relax your stomach when you exhale.

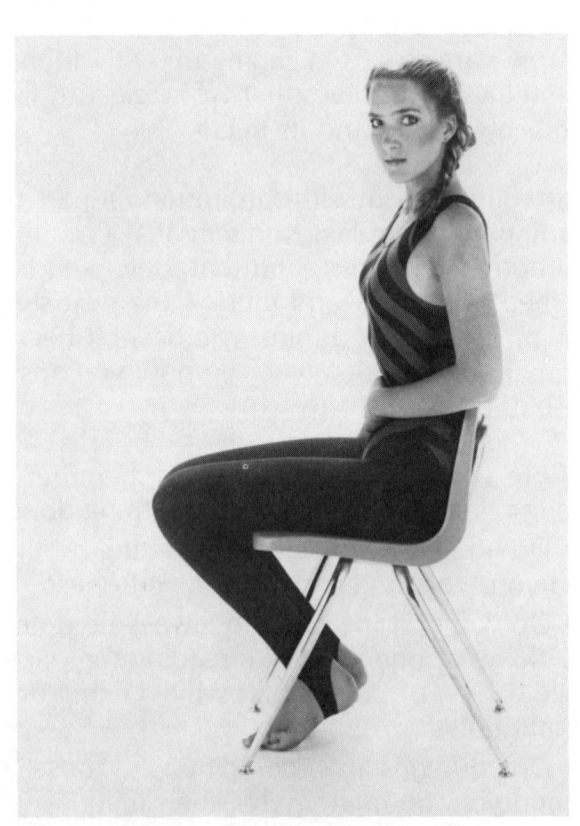

When you inhale, suck in your stomach.

- Do you find other people's affairs "none of your business"?
- Do you feel guilty when you relax?

If you had to answer "yes" to a lot of these questions, then you would be wise to think about changing your current pattern of living to include a little self-motivated relaxation. Your life, as it stands now, is laden with stress. And although there seem to be a million things more important than relaxing, well, *you* are still the most important person in your own life, and if you don't stop to take care of yourself, then probably no one else will either. And if you don't stop to think about your own needs every once in a while, you won't be in any condition to worry about anything else.

QUIET TIME

Getting in touch with yourself is sometimes as easy as sitting down in a nice, quiet place and shutting your eyes for a few minutes. I think it's

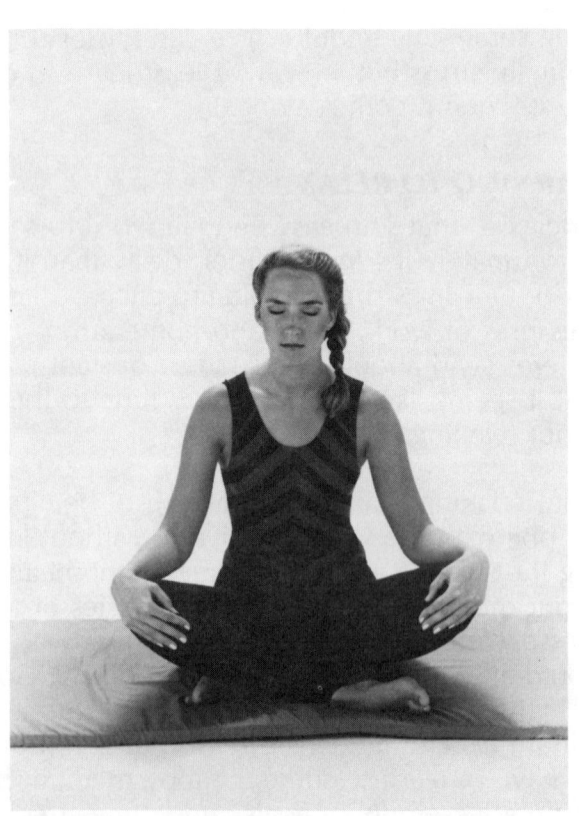

A great position for relaxation, legs crossed, hands on knees.

very important for each one of you to have your own space, your own time to reflect and think about the events of the day, or to just wash the events of the day out of your system.

Set aside a time each day for quiet reflection, whether it be during a break at work, or in the evening when the pressures of the day are absent. You don't have to take a relaxation class and fork out a lot of money to learn how to make some time for yourself — just do it! Ten or fifteen minutes won't impede your busy schedule one bit, and you'll feel so much better for making time for yourself. This will help you to deal with stress on a day-to-day basis, and can even make you a happier person in the long run.

- Sit down in a comfortable chair and kick off your shoes. Make sure the room is relatively quiet; sometimes having the room darkened is even more relaxing. There is something about following the pattern of one's own breathing that is very relaxing. Don't try to suppress thoughts — just let them flow in and out of your subconscious. Remain quiet and calm for about ten minutes, if you can. You'll be surprised at the effect this has on your mind and body.

- Pull the curtains and lie down on the bed. Starting at the top of your head, try to relax every muscle in your body. Pretend the tension in your body is melting into the bed. Move from one part of your body to another, telling that particular body area to relax. Once you have reached your feet, remain motionless for a few minutes and let your body enjoy being worry-free. This exercise can be so relaxing that some people fall asleep before they've finished.

- Put on your favorite album, preferably soft, easy music, and just sit on the floor for a few minutes, absorbing the mood of the music. Then do a few deep stretches. Make your movements slow and deliberate, working to the rhythm of the music. Run through the stretches in your exercise warm-up routine, but doing each as though you were moving in slow motion. This helps to relax the muscles and relieve some of the tension that can accompany a stressful day.

- For a change, try eating dinner without the television set on. If you are dining with others, light a few candles and dim the lights. Candlelight dinners should not be reserved exclusively for romantic encounters; candles set a relaxing tone any time, any day of the week. And instead of retiring in front of the tube for the night, put on some music, or pick up a book and read (for pleasure only!). Simple habits like these are the nicest ways to escape the pressures and stresses of the day.

GETTING OUT

Many times, when something is really bothering you, just getting away from that particular situation for a few minutes will help to ward off the stress that readily accumulates in your body. You can apply this principle in both your professional and personal life. If you have a hectic work environment, never, never hesitate to take your breaks. It may seem like frivolous activity on the surface, but those breaks are allowed for good reason. Breaks are a time to relax, to socialize, to grab a snack or just to spend some time alone getting yourself together. Make sure you don't turn your breaks into eat fests, however.

Similarly, your lunch hour should be your own time, and, if possible, make every effort to get out of your immediate work environment during that time. Give yourself a chance to get away from it all. To really make the most of a lunch hour, you might bring a bag lunch to work and then take a walk to a nearby park to dine. Walking will give you the exercise your body needs, and getting out of the office to a pretty place like a park will be a pleasant diversion from the strains of work.

If most of your time is spent at home with little ones, try to do the same. Perhaps you can put the baby in a stroller, pack a picnic lunch for yourself and walk to a favorite place in the neighborhood. Children enjoy time to themselves almost as much as we do, especially when they are very young. If you really feel adventurous, pack your baby or toddler into a stroller and go out for a jog. Many women find that this is a great way to get some exercise and relax at the same time. And don't feel self-conscious! Your neighbors will admire your ingenuity.

FEELING GOOD

Remember, your body and your mind work on the same wavelength. What affects your mind will affect your body, and vice versa.

Well, those effects don't necessarily have to be negative. Treating your body with care and gentleness will have positive effects on your mind; and, similarly, treating your body to the some kindness every once in a while tends to make you feel much better all over. Often, when stresses hit, we neglect our bodies. Paying attention to it just might eliminate the negative effects.

Besides vigorous exercise, which is the best way to help your body handle stress, there are lots of ways that you can make your body feel needed and more at ease:

- When was the last time you took a long, hot bath — just for the sake of taking a bath? If you can't remember, then now might be the right time to experience the calming affects that warm water can have on the body. Lace the bath water with a little sea salt or bath oil, for an extra pampering for your skin. Enjoy the warmth of the water.

- Have you ever had a massage? If you have, you know the wonderful consequences that massage can have on the body. Treat yourself to a massage on occasion. If you have the time and the money, visit a professional masseuse or masseur, and experience the many different types of massage. If not, have your husband, boyfriend or friend work out the kinks in your muscles and joints by gently kneading and stroking the skin on your back, thighs, arms and neck.

- Restricting what you eat can help to relieve the stress on your body. Lots of refined sugar and caffeine-laden foods can give you the jitters, and can increase and intensify the effects of stress on the body. When you are feeling especially low, try a glass of warm milk with a little brown sugar. It will help to soothe your stomach and give you a more restful sleep.

- Calculate your mood as far as food is concerned. If your mood is particularly crotchety, don't pork out on a lot of rich foods. Your system will have a hard time digesting it (remember, the fight or flight response triggers the digestive processes to slow down); besides, the reason you are eating is probably because you are feeling down, and that's a poor excuse to take in calories. If you feel low, try some hot soup or a cup of herb or cinnamon tea. Let your foods be healing, not hurting.

EVERYBODY NEEDS A TEDDY BEAR

Remember when you were little? If you were feeling bad, if things just weren't going your way, you could always count on teddy to see you through. Hugging that teddy bear always seemed to make things so much better — it was so nice to have something to soak up all those salty tears.

People don't change all that much from childhood, and though we may have grown taller and possibly wiser, we all need the comfort we experienced as children. Perhaps that comfort does not come in the form of a teddy bear anymore: Now it might be a good friend, an endearing hobby or a special place. Whatever that comfort might be, don't deny yourself the opportunity to enjoy the peacefulness that goes with having a "teddy bear."

Give yourself an outlet for your frustrations, just don't take it out on teddy bear. For many, the best way to vent frustrations is through vigorous activity — like running, weight training or aerobic dance. But you can find comfort through other means. If you have a favorite hobby, such as painting, woodworking or cooking, allow yourself to get completely immersed in that activity every now and then. It will add diversity to your life as well as give you a chance to think about something other than your trials and tribulations.

Similarly, problems seem much less formidable and terrible when you can talk them out with someone who cares about you. While people can be the primary cause of our problems, they can also be a major source of comfort. Don't bottle your problems up inside you. Seek out a good, understanding friend, and ask for advice. Or just ask her to listen. Often, just getting a problem off your chest alleviates a lot of the stress that can accompany that problem.

TAKE A BREAK!

I had been feeling particularly bad one month. Work was awful; all of my responsibilities had piled up, my superiors were not delighted with my performance and what I was getting done lacked character, thought and dedication. The headaches that plagued me in college had returned, and my stomach was a candidate for a Pepto-Bismol ad. Even the little things in my life were affected: I couldn't balance my checkbook properly, and even making my bed and taking a shower were dreaded chores. Worst of all, I was taking all of my anger and frustration, which had grown completely out of proportion, on the people I loved the most. And that hurt.

Luckily, I was saved. We had planned to take a vacation that month; nothing elaborate, just a trip into the mountains for some hiking and general relaxing. And I guess it was just the thing I needed — a few days in the fresh air, exploring new places I'd never seen and enjoying the gifts of nature. It made me slow down, relax and put everything back into perspective. I forgot about all the tensions at work, and when I finally did let them enter my mind again, I was calm enough to be able to evaluate the situations and come up with workable solutions to all my problems. I had come down from the mountains feeling refreshed and rejuvenated, and ready to tackle the world once again.

The moral of this little story is: Everybody needs a break now and then. The stresses and strains of everyday life can really take their toll on us, whether we're housewives or electrical engineers, school teachers or politicians. And one of the best remedies you can administer to yourself is a nice, simple vacation. It doesn't have to be a magnificent extravaganza; you don't have to jet to Tahiti or take a world cruise. Just do something — a drive to your favorite lookout on top of a hill for a few hours of contemplation, or a stroll on the beach.

Take the time to get away from it all, and don't make excuses. I know one woman who skips her vacation each year because, she says, she has too much to do. "I don't have time for vacations. I've got kids and a husband and all kinds of responsibilities. What would they do without me?" Well, chances are they would do just fine without her, and they'd probably enjoy being around her more if she did take the time to get away for a while. If your place of employment allows vacations, for heaven's sake, take advantage of them. That's what they're for. Managers realize that vacations can be therapeutic for their employees and for themselves, too.

So go ahead and give yourself that extra time to unwind and enjoy a carefree couple of days — or hours. Here are some of my favorite activities that make vacation time unforgettable, relaxing and not too expensive.

• Go camping with a friend. Whether you head to the mountains, the plains or the desert, camping provides a way to relax and see the beauty of nature all at the same time. Your trip can be as cheap or as expensive as you wish — and don't forget your fishin' pole.

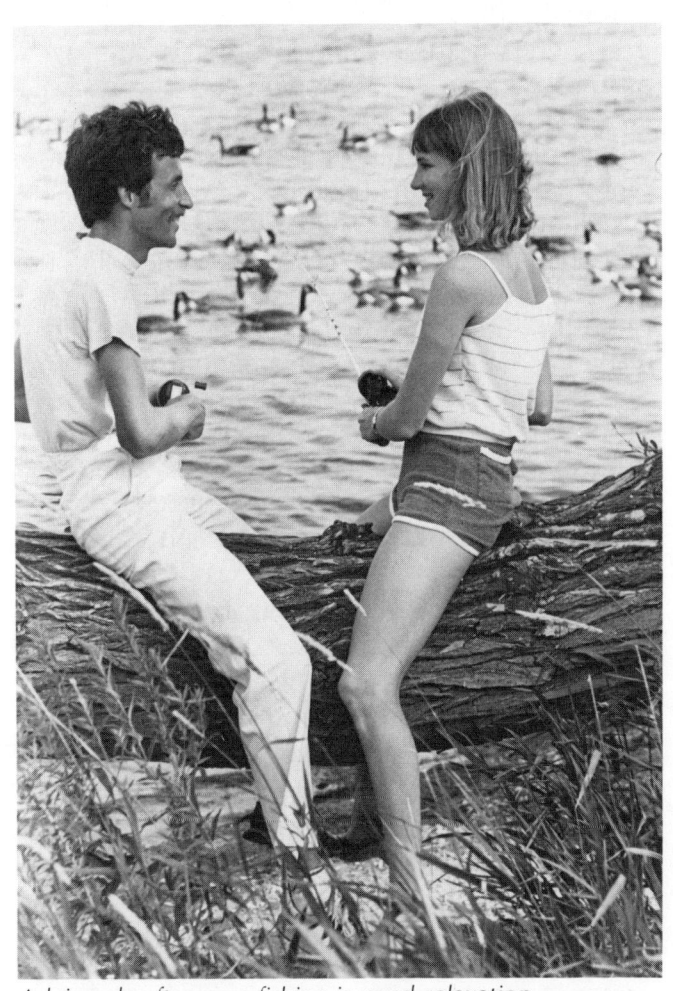

A leisurely afternoon fishing is good relaxation.

- How about a relaxing day hike? You don't have to spend lots of money on expensive camping equipment and campsite reservations; just hop in your car, or better yet, hop on your bicycle, and head to your favorite spot. Perhaps it's a stretch of wooded parkland, or a secluded beach. Sometimes it's nice to bring a friend along so you can share some of the more memorable moments of your trek. Other times, you might want the peace of mind that comes from being by yourself. The only requirement for this "mini-vacation" is a pair of quality walking shoes.

- Have you ever gone canoeing? It's great fun, and if you get to do some paddling, it's good exercise, too. And what a great way to discover new worlds: gliding down a peaceful, quiet river. Canoe rentals are generally very reasonable, and if you can locate one on your own, perhaps from a good friend, bring the friend along and it won't cost you a dime. Canoeing is a great way to get your mind off the cares of your world and focused on the beauty of the rest of the world.

- There's nothing quite like the pampering and fussing you get when you stay at a quaint little bed-and-breakfast inn. You know, the kind where old Mrs. Smith does all the cooking; where all the rooms have their own four-poster beds and fireplaces; where the bathtub sits on little claw feet and fills up to your neck. Prices for bed-and-breakfast (called so because most often the price for a night includes a breakfast in bed as well) country inns range from very cheap to very expensive, so there's bound to be one that fits right into your budget. To find out more about country inns in your area, get in touch with your chamber of commerce, or the city or town council. There might be a place waiting right around the corner from you.

- Sometimes, getting in your car and taking a drive can be one of the most relaxing things in the world. Turn on some nice music and just let yourself go. (Be careful, though: Don't try something like this if you are very upset, or if you have been trying to drink a bad spell out of your system. Many traffic accidents and fatalities occur for this very reason.) Perhaps you might want to bring a friend along to talk to. Stop at out-of-the-way places during your travels; visit shops and parks that you normally pass by; slow down and look at the country around you.

BEWARE OF CRUTCHES

Nobody is going to preach to you, in this book, about the hazards of smoking cigarettes, drinking alcohol or taking drugs (recreational drugs, that is). It is assumed that you are a person who has made a commitment to a fit lifestyle and that you are already aware of those dangers.

But just remember one more thing about relaxing: It is something that has to be done from within, not from without. Drinking or smoking, by themselves, are not the issue here, although an issue could be made for each subject, that would take up several books of this size. The issue is why you drink, smoke or partake of drugs. If you do so to relax — often — then you are looking for trouble.

Drinking or smoking will not relax you without also creating dependency. These bad habits may offer you a sense of security for a while, but this false feeling wears off quickly. In order to regain that comforting feeling, you will have to pour yourself another drink, or light up another cigarette. In short, those activities become crutches and when you are feeling tense and under pressure, you turn to them in hopes that they will carry you through your troubles. The more you turn to them in time of need, the stronger your dependence on them becomes.

Use your head, don't use a crutch. If you find that you are turning to things like smoking and drinking in order to relax, you may want to sit down and have a talk with someone you can trust, whether it's your doctor, a good friend or a counselor. Find out why you feel the need to pursue these activities for relaxation, and together perhaps the two of you can come up with alternate solutions to your problems. Let your mind and your body be self-sufficient.

WHAT THOSE PILLS DO TO YOU

AMPHETAMINES	SEDATIVE HYPNOTICS
Stimulants • amphetamine (e.g. Benzedrine*) • dextro-amphetamine (e.g. Dexedrine*) • methamphetamine (e.g. Neodrine*) • phenmetrazine (e.g. Preludin*)	**Barbiturates** • amobarbital (e.g. Amytal*) • secobarbital (e.g. Seconal*) • pentobarbital (e.g. Nembutal*) **Non-Barbiturates** • ethchlorvynol (e.g. Placidyl*) • flurazepam (e.g. Dalmane*) • glutethimide (e.g. Doriden*)
Short-term Effects • reduced appetite • increased energy and postponement of fatigue • increased alertness • faster breathing • increased heart rate and blood pressure, which leads to increased risk of burst blood vessels or heart failure • dilation of pupils **With Larger Doses** • talkativeness, restlessness, excitation • sense of power and superiority • illusions and hallucinations frequently occur • some frequent users become irritable, aggressive, paranoid, panicky or violent • high blood pressure, dry mouth, fever, sweating and sleeplessness	**Short-term Effects** • small dose relieves anxiety and tension, producing calmness and muscular relaxation • a somewhat larger dose produces effects similar to those of alcohol intoxication — a high feeling, slurred speech, staggering • produces sleep in a quiet setting • much larger doses produce unconsciousness • acute overdose can be fatal because of suppression of breathing • increase the effects of alcohol, opiates, minor tranquilzers
Long-term Effects • malnutrition • increased susceptibility to infections • tolerance with high doses • psychological dependence • after stopping, a long sleep, depression and ravenous appetite usually occur.	**Long-term Effects** • tolerance and dependence develop rapidly if large doses used • sedative hypnotics do not produce completely normal sleep; user may feel tired and irritable even though a sleeping state occurs • upon withdrawal, temporary sleep disturbances occur. This may lead the user to incorrectly decide that more of the drug is required • abrupt withdrawal leads to progressive restlessness, anxiety and possibly delirium, convulsions and death
Legal Status • these drugs may be obtained only through prescription	**Legal Status** • these drugs may be obtained only through prescription

*Registered trademarks

MINOR TRANQUILIZERS	ANTIHISTAMINES
Depressants • meprobamate (e.g. Equanil*) • diazepam (e.g. Valium*, Vivol*) • chlordiazepoxide (Librium*)	**Hay Fever and Cold Preparations** • diphenhydramine (e.g. Benadryl*) • chlorpheniramine (e.g. Chlor-Tripolon*) • phenyltoloxamine (e.g. Sinutab*) • promethazine (e.g. Phenergan*) • many other types and brand names
Short-term Effects • calms hyperactivity, tension and agitation • diminished emotional responses to external stimuli, for example, pain • muscle relaxation • reduced alertness • gives short-term relief of anxiety • combats severe withdrawal effects of other depressant drugs • with larger doses, possible impairment of muscle co-ordination, dizziness, low blood pressure and/or fainting • increases effects of alcohol, sedatives and opiates	**Short-term Effects** • decreased nasal congestion, discharge, rashes • some types reduce motion sickness or nausea • most are fairly potent local anesthetics (can cause numbness of tongue) • drowsiness, uncoordination, fatigue • increase the effects of sedative-hypnotics, alcohol, minor tranquilizers • may cause excitement, tremor, hallucinations, fever, dilated pupils in children and in some adults • may occasionally trigger seizures in epileptics
Long-term Effects • physical dependence • withdrawal reaction like that of sedative hypnotics	**Long-term Effects** • prolonged use occasionally *causes* allergy instead of relieving it • rarely suppress formation of white blood cells • can cause deformity in babies if taken by pregnant women
Legal Status • these drugs may be obtained only through prescription	**Legal Status** • some preparations can be bought without prescription in pharmacies • stronger preparations available by prescription only

Reprinted with permission from the Alcoholism and Drug Addiction Research Foundation.

5 APPEARANCE

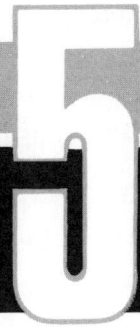

POLISHING UP: KEEPING YOURSELF LOOKING GREAT

Beauty: One of the Best Reasons to Get Fit

As you apply your makeup, think about all the reasons you decided to dedicate a little of your time and energy to becoming fit and healthy. The justifications for health and fitness are endless. But while proper nourishment of your body's cells and protecting yourself against disease and illness are very valid reasons for embarking on a program of fitness, they probably weren't the ones that motivated you in the first place. More often than not, vanity plays the biggest role in convincing a woman to adopt more healthful ways.

Why? Because women always want to be more beautiful than they are, and many of them find it through fitness. It's no secret. One of the great fringe benefits of being fit and healthy is a new kind of beauty born of vitality. All the makeup in the world can't emulate it. And the reason that many women look to fitness is to find tha beauty, to become more attractive, to look good outside as well as feel good inside.

Beauty, of course, isn't only skin-deep, but the kind of beauty that most of us search for all our lives is. This section is about the beauty that is skin-deep, and the ways through which you can accentuate the natural, glowing beauty that goes along with fitness.

SKIN TALK

Take a good long look in the mirror. What's the very first thing you set your gaze upon? It's your face, of course. Or more accurately, it's the skin on your face. Look at it again. What do you see? Is that face in the mirror the picture of loveliness? Is that skin fresh-looking and soft? Or is it less than what you might imagine it could be? Is it pale and lifeless, or have those nasty little age lines begun to show up around your eyes, nose and corners of your mouth?

Chances are that your face is never quite what you want it to be. Or the rest of your skin, for that matter. But if you're going to make a commitment to fitness, you might as well take a little extra care with your skin. After all, skin is the most visible part of your body, and you can tell a lot about a person's overall health by noting the condition of her skin.

Before we get involved in lengthy conversations about skin beauty and lotions and potions, let's back up a bit and talk about some basics. First, what is skin? Well, believe it or not, your skin is an organ; it performs duties just like your heart or your brain. And skin has the honor of being the largest organ of your body. The average-sized woman has about one and one-half yards of skin covering her body, at an average weight of about seven pounds. Underneath that skin is a layer of fat, called subcutaneous fat, which weighs about thirty-five

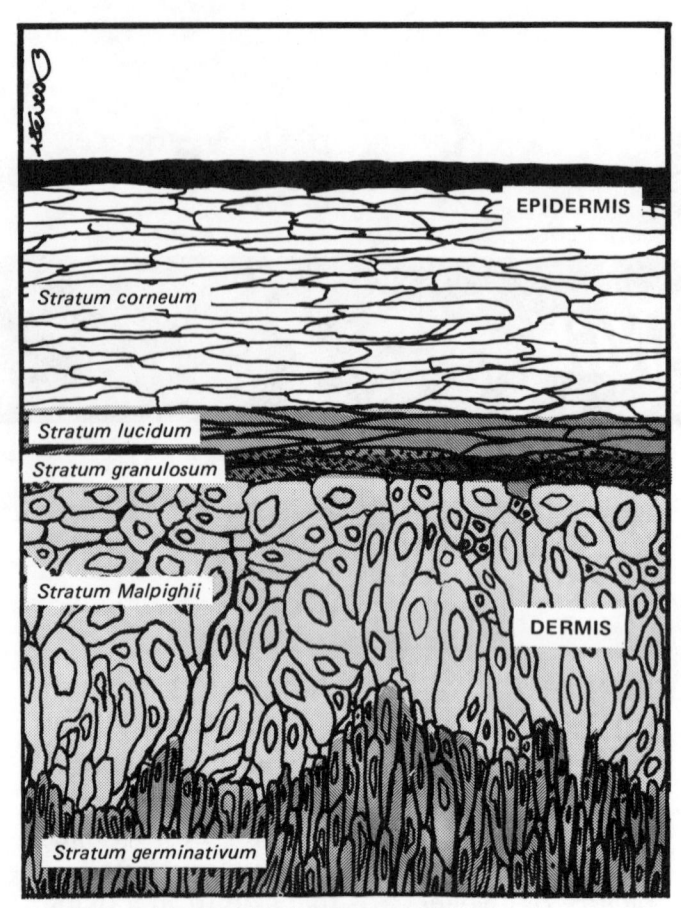

Cross-section showing layers of the skin.

pounds altogether. For most women, that's about one-quarter of their total body weight; you probably would never have guessed that. And skin may vary in thickness — from one-fiftieth of an inch on your delicate eyelids to one-eighth, possibly even one-quarter inch on the palms of your hands and the tough soles of your feet.

Your skin is composed of two basic layers: the epidermis, which is the outer layer that you can see and touch, and the dermis, the inner layer where all the work takes place. Beneath the dermis is a thick layer of fat, the subcutaneous fat, that separates the skin from the rest of the tissue in your body. The lower portion of the epidermis is called the Malpighian layer. This is where the miracle of skin reproduction occurs.

At the base of this Malpighian layer, cells are continually dividing to form new cells. As this multiplication occurs, the new cells are pushed to the surface of the skin, where they eventually harden, flatten out and are sloughed off.

Thus, the outer layer of your skin is always laden with a lot of dead cells. But don't be alarmed; cleansing and rubbing helps remove this dead layer of cells.

Even as you read this, your skin is dying and rejuvenating itself. The cells in the Malpighian layer divide approximately once every hour, and it takes approximately five days for the whole process, from cell birth to cell death, to take place.

The hard surface of your skin is the responsibility of a material called keratin. Keratin is largely made up of protein, and it forms in granules in the cells of the epidermis. This substance helps to keep your skin waterproofed; notice, during a rain, that the wetness may seep through your clothes, but, happily, not any farther than the surface of your skin. The sebaceous glands in the skin also help to protect the skin from water. They produce a thin barrier of oil that seals impurities out and retains the skin's natural moisture. When the skin is exposed to very cold weather, or if you soak in a tub too long, this oily barrier is washed away, leaving your skin vulnerable to dryness. More about dryness later.

Since your skin is an organ made up of cells, as in the rest of your body, it has to be properly nourished. This nourishment, in the form of oxygen and nutrients that have been broken down by digestion, is fed to the skin by a delicate network of tiny blood vessels in the dermis. Minute branches of this network, capillaries, extend up to the surface to feed the epidermis. After the skin is "fed," the blood removes wastes that accumulate in the skin — all in a matter of micro-seconds, of course.

Also nourished by that intricate blood vessel network are the glands, which are located in the dermis. Basically, there are two types of glands: the sweat glands and the sebaceous glands, which were described earlier. The sebaceous glands produce sebum, that thin, oily barrier, which contains fatty materials called lipids. This substance lubricates the skin and protects it from dryness. Sebum also acts as a catch-all for the by-products of cell reproduction, namely the dead skin cells.

You have some three million sweat glands all over your body. Each gland is a little coiled tube surrounded by a profusion of tiny blood vessels; it looks kind of like a curlicued ribbon from a Christmas package. This tube extends through the epidermis and empties out onto the skin's surface. The sweat that pours out from the gland and onto your skin carries with it waste and impurities, and sweating helps to regulate body temperature as well.

HOW WE BECOME LITTLE OLD LADIES BEFORE WE SHOULD

You would think that with all of that activity taking place under and on the surface of the skin that we might possibly be able to retain the soft, radiant and rosy skin we were all born with. Why, then, does our skin become weathered and wrinkled as time marches on?

The system working within our skin is a nearly perfect system, but, unfortunately, we do not live in a perfect environment — as far as our skin is concerned, anyway. Our skin is under constant attack by both visible and invisible forces that, unless we mount a counterattack against them, will gradually take their toll. This toll we know as aging.

Scientists and research have found that "actinic radiation," or that part of the electromagnetic spectrum that can damage skin cells, is the factor that contributes most to what they have termed "premature aging."

The sun is the main culprit, as it is the source of the actinic radiation that damages our skin. Here's what happens: The actinic rays affect the fibroblasts — cells that form collagen and elastic tissue. The result is the formation of abnormal cells whose function is altered. You might not be able to notice the changes at first, but sooner or later, the effects of actinic radiation will become apparent: Skin elasticity diminishes; the epidermis thins and loses its ability to retain water, leading to dryness; subcutaneous fat diminishes; and blood vessels decrease in numbers. Eventually, your skin will become dry, cracked and wrinkled.

This same actinic radiation can be responsible for causing certain skin cancers. The rays damage the nuclei of your skin cells, which causes them to deform. These deformed cells then divide to create more abnormal cells, which in turn may result in a cancerous growth. Women with fair skin are particularly prone to skin damage because their skin lacks the pigment melanin, which helps to scatter these rays and lessen their effect on the cells. If you have fair skin, it is wise to be careful not to expose your skin too long or too frequently to the sun.

So our skin is doomed from the start, right? Well, aging is a process we cannot stop, but it is one that we can postpone and dilute, if we practice a preventive skin-care routine. Good skin care involves three things: cleansing, moisturizing and exercising. Let's look at each separately.

Cleansing — Remember when your mother scolded you for not washing your hands before dinner, or for missing that dreaded area behind your ears? Well, Mother always knows best: Cleansing your skin is an important part of skin care, for children and for adults.

This was not always so. Our ancestors believed that bathing was akin to witchcraft, and that the Lord would strike them down dead if they attempted to get clean. So they didn't. Even the lovely virgin Queen Elizabeth I of England left bathing out of her beauty routine (It is rumored that more than an inch of makeup had accumulated on her face by the time of her death!)

We of the modern world seem to have struck out in the opposite direction. We employ soaps, antiperspirants, mouthwashes, toothpastes and every kind of product imaginable to scrub our bodies squeaky clean — almost too clean, in fact. Proper cleansing is a must; it helps to remove dirt and oils from the surface of the skin, wipes away the dead skin cells produced from skin rejuvenation, and helps to stimulate the skin's circulation. But how much does it take to do all that? Not as much as we think.

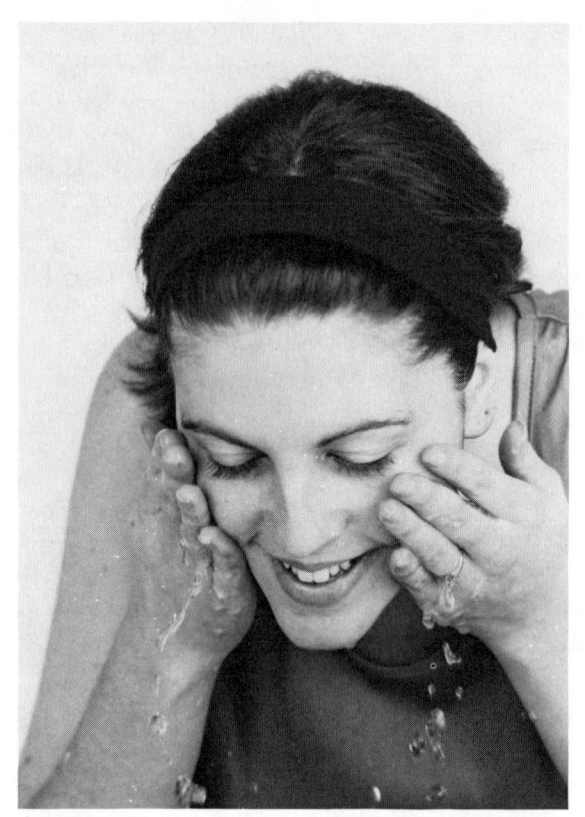

Water is the magic ingredient in face cleansing.

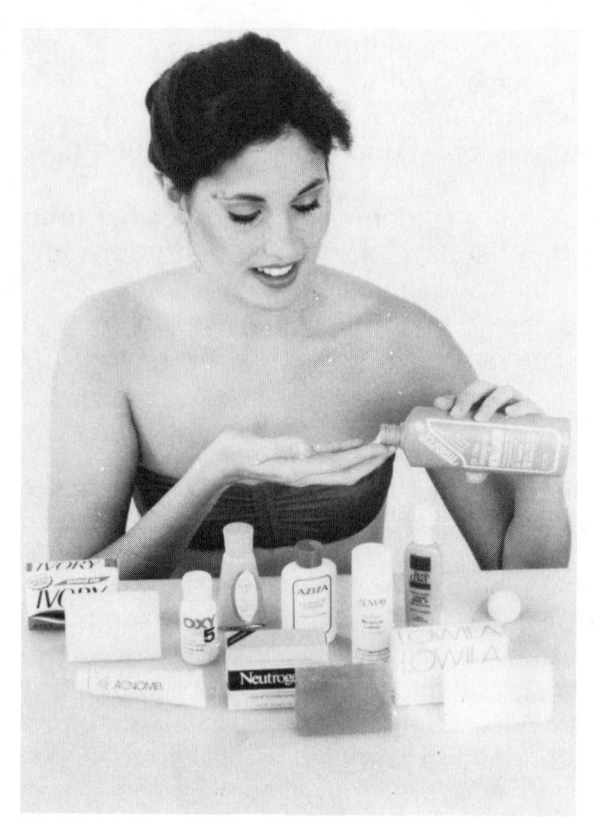

Facial products range from moisturizers to makeup.

Let's first look at basic soap. Soap is an emulsifier; that is, it makes oil and dirt on the skin's surface water-soluble so that it can be washed away in a shower or bath. Sounds good so far. The problem with soap is that in order for it to do its job, it has to be alkaline, and this alkalinity can have some fairly detrimental effects on our slightly acidic skin. Not only does soap wash away dirt and dead skin cells, but many times its strong cleansing action can sap the skin of the essential natural oils it needs to stay moist and soft. You may have noticed that after bathing or showering with soap, your skin feels tight and drawn. That's because of the soap.

Some skin types tolerate this harsh cleansing action of soap better than others, but all faces suffer. Facial skin is much more delicate and sensitive to dryness; therefore, it is best to consider another type of cleansing agent.

Perhaps a cleansing cream or lotion would be best for your facial skin. In fact, most cosmetologists recommend that you use a cleanser milder than soap for all of your bathing. Most cleansing creams have some oil, and are washed off with water or swabbed off with tissue or cotton balls. If you tend to have very dry skin, this type of cleanser might be best for you.

If you're not sure what to use on your skin, or if you have problem, dry or oily skin, it's best to check with a dermatologist or cosmetologist before you decide. But, generally speaking, tone down on the soap. Our bodies are not as dirty as we think; sometimes using a loofah sponge or washcloth with plain water will be enough to remove most dirt and oils. be surprised at how ''clean'' you feel, and your skin will thank you.

Moisturizing — Moisturizing means putting moisture back into the skin. That's a fairly easy definition to swallow, but because there are so many products on the market that claim to be the best moisturizer you can buy, many women are confused about just which one to choose.

Let's first go back and review a little of the skin's anatomy. Your skin is composed primarily of water — about 70 percent. Most of that water, however, lies in the inner layer, or dermis, of the skin. The outer layer, or epidermis, contains only about 10 percent water, which makes it very vulnerable to dryness. The epidermis does contain little sponges, called hygroscopic particles, that help to hold the molecules of water in your skin, but without extra help, moisture evaporates very easily from the surface of the skin.

This is where the sebaceous glands come into play. That oil they produce forms a thin barrier on your skin's surface, which aids in retarding moisture evaporation and gives your skin its sheen and softness. This is a nearly perfect system, where oil and water mix quite nicely.

Once again, the problem is that our skin doesn't live in an absolutely perfect environment. Nature's elements, like wind, rain, cold weather and sunlight, combined with lots of conscientious bathing and showering, strip away that oily barrier. And, once again, the skin is subject to drying.

That's where your moisturizer helps out. Basically, all moisturizers are a blend of oil and water; some of the water in the preparation sinks into the epidermis, plumping up those thirsty cells, while the oil remains on the surface of your skin, providing an artificial barrier against evaporation and making it smooth and soft.

But which to choose? As a fit, healthy woman, you want to use the very best moisturizer for your skin, and with so many bottles and jars of creams and lotions taunting you from department store shelves, it's easy to get confused. Take comfort in this, though: Most commercial preparations do just about the same thing. It's the proportion of water to oil in the mixture that makes one look and feel different from another. Many dermatologists claim that the best moisturizer for dry skin is plain old Vaseline petroleum jelly applied to the skin when it is moist, such as right after a nice, hot bath. But none of us want to walk the streets with a face full of Vaseline.

The important thing to remember about moisturizer is not necessarily what you apply, but when you apply it. Dabbing on your cream or smoothing on your lotion at the proper time will maximize the healing benefits that the moisturizer can offer.

The best time, say dermatologists, for your moisturizing routine is right after bathing or showering. The skin is moist and plump because it has soaked up (thanks to those hygroscopic sponges) some of the water on its surface. Even if your skin is not overly dry, it is a good idea to moisturize after every shower or bath. It will help to keep your skin soft and supple, and protect it from the dryness that leads to premature aging.

If your skin is oily to normal, you probably should use a preparation that doesn't contain a lot of oil. Lotions that are water-based or that flow easily when poured into your hand are your best bet. If your skin is on the dry side, use a cream; creams contain considerably more oil, and will give you the added moisture you need.

Some women wonder about using night creams. Night creams are fine, if your skin needs them, but generally, a good skin-care and moisturizing routine during the day will reduce the need to load your skin up with heavy substances at night. Nighttime is a time to let your skin breathe a little bit; unless it has been recommended for use by a dermatologist or skin-care specialist, you probably don't need one.

The ABCs of Skin-Care Products

Still confused about what to use? Sometimes knowing just exactly what manufacturers put into those bottles and jars helps you make your moisturizer choice. Here's a list of some common moisturizing and skin-cleansing ingredients, and a short explanation of what those foreign substances do on your skin (some of these ingredients are also contained in shampoos, which will be discussed later):

Acetylated Lanolin a moisturizing agent derived from lanolin (see lanolin).
Algin a stabilizing agent derived from seaweed.
Allantoin an antibacterial compound that has skin-soothing and softening properties. It is found in a lot of moisturizers.
Amphoteric 2 a mild cleansing agent.
Benzalkonium chloride an agent that acts upon the surface of the skin; usually included in cleansers as a preservative.

Benzethonium chloride a surface-acting agent that is responsible for dispersing and wetting action; it is another preservative.
2-Bromo-2 nitropropane-1.3-diol this mouthful is nothing but another preservative.
Cetyl alcohol also called palmityl alcohol, this is a fatty alcohol derived from animal or vegetable sources; it is commonly used as an emulsifying agent.
Chloroxynol an antibacterial compound.
Cholesterol a component of skin secretions used in skin-care products as an emollient, or moisturizing agent.
Choleth 24 a water-soluble form of cholesterol that is also used as a moisturizing agent.
Cinozate a sunscreen.
Citric acid a naturally occuring organic acid found in citrus fruits and used to adjust the pH balance of various products.
Cocamide DEA a derivative of coconut oil used in cleansers and shampoos to increase viscosity, or thickness, of a product, and to stabilize foam.
Cocamidopropyl betaine another cleansing agent derived from coconut oil.
D&C red No. 19 a FDA approved substance that produces a pinkish red color.
D&C violet No. 2 a deep purple color approved for cosmetic use.
DEA lauraminopropionate a cleanser.
Disopropyl adipate an oil-soluble substance that produces the "oily-without-feeling-greasy" feel on your skin.
Dimethicone a silicone derivative used to promote silkiness of the skin and to form a thin, protective barrier.
Dimethoxane a preservative.
Dipropylene glycol a water-soluble substance that gives a slick, oily feel without being greasy.
FD&C blue, green, reds and yellows coloring agents approved for cosmetic use by the FDA.
Glycerin another moisturizing agent that gives lubrication to the skin without making it feel greasy.
Glyceryl stearate a surface-cleansing agent used as an emulsion stabilizer.
Hexylene glycol a substance included in some bubble-bath formulas to thin them out.
Hydrolyzed animal protein a form of protein that can act as a moisturizer and a conditioner.
Hydroxypropyl cellulose a substance used as an emulsifier, stabilizer and thickener in some cosmetic preparations.

Isopropyl lanolate a lanolin derivative used as a moisturizing agent.
Isostearyl alcohol a lightweight, non-greasy compound used in cosmetics to promote a silky feel.
Kaolin a substance that binds water and is used to stabilize emulsions.
Lanolin this is wool grease that has been cleaned and purified but not chemically modified. It contains no water and is thick and sticky. It's used as a moisturizing agent.
Lanolin oil the liquid portion of cleaned and purified lanolin; added to cosmetic preparations as a moisturizing agent.
Lecithen the acts as an emulsifier, preservative and moisturizing agent. It works well in combination with other formulas, promoting penetration of the skin.
Methylparaben a preservative.
Mineral oil a light, purified petroleum oil that gives the skin a protective layer through which moisture cannot evaporate.
Ozokerite a wax used to stiffen the consistency of cosmetic preparations.
Petrolatum a jellylike oil that prevents moisture evaporation from the skin's surface.
Polysorbate 20 and 60 helps to make perfume oils soluble in water.
Propylene glycol a common moisturizing agent derived from natural gas.
Propylparaben a preservative.
Sodium lauraminopropionate a mild surface-cleansing agent.
Sodium lauryl sulfate used as a cleanser in shampoos; also an emulsifying aid.
Sodium myreth sulfate another cleanser.
Sodium stearate an emulsifying aid.
Sorbitol corn sugar that is used as a moisturizing agent.
Stearic acid a fatty acid used in cosmetic emulsions.
TEA (triethanolamine) an excellent emulsifier; combines with fatty acids to form surface-cleansing agents.
Zinc oxide used to make products opaque; also a sun block.

Don't let all those chemical names scare you! A lot of people would have you believe that anything made with "chemicals" couldn't possibly be good for your skin. Well, if you think about it, everything in this world is made of chemicals, including our bodies. The idea that synthetically produced chemicals are any worse for you than naturally occurring ones just doesn't hold water. There isn't any evidence to prove that cosmetics made with "all-natural" ingredients are any more effective, or any less harmful, than synthetics, at least as far as your skin is concerned. As one dermatologist so aptly put it, "Poison ivy is natural, too, but you wouldn't want to go putting that on your skin."

This doesn't mean that you shouldn't use products whose labels do read "natural" ingredients. Many natural substances, like sesame, avocado and safflower oils as well as vitamins and minerals, combine to make excellent skin-care products. It's just that, basically, prove that cosmetics made with "all-natural" ingredients are any more effective, or any less

There are a few substances to be wary of, however. Check the labels on your products carefully, and try to avoid using the ones that contain these chemicals:

Ammonium chloride — This is an ammonium salt that occurs naturally. It is colorless and odorless, and is used as an acidifier in permanent wave solutions, eye lotions, and as a cooling and stimulating skin wash. It is also used industrially in freezing mixtures, batteries, dyes, and safety explosives, and in medicine as a urinary acidifier and a diuretic. If ingested, it can cause nausea, vomiting and acidosis, and as with any ammonia solution, concentrated solution can be very irritating to your skin.

Balsam Peru — This is a dark brown, viscous liquid with a pleasant odor that's used in face masks, perfumes, cream hair rinses and astringents. Obtained from Peruvian balsam in Central America near the Pacific Coast, this substance is irritating to the skin and may cause contact dermatitis and a stuffy nose.

Formaldehyde — This substance is as foreboding as its name suggests. A colorless gas obtained by the oxidation of methyl alcohol, it is used in nail hardeners, nail polish, soap and hair-growing products. Ingestion can cause severe abdominal pain, internal bleeding, loss of ability to urinate, vertigo, coma and death. Skin reactions to formaldehyde are very common, since the chemical can be both irritating and allergy-causing. Products to prevent nails from chipping and peeling often contain formaldehyde, and physicians have reported severe reactions to such nail hardeners, including discoloration, bleeding around the nail, dryness and even loss of nails. The cuticle and surrounding skin have also been affected.

Ethylenediamine Tetraacetic Acid (EDTA) — An important compound in many cosmetics, this substance is used as a sequestering agent, particularly in shampoos. It may be irritating to the skin and the mucous membranes and can cause allergies like skin rashes.

Boric Acid — An antiseptic with bactericidal and fungicidal properties, this substance is used in baby powders, eye creams, liquid powders, mouthwashes, protective creams, after-shave lotions, soaps and skin fresheners. It is still widely used in commercial preparations despite repeated warnings from the American Medical Association as to its possible toxicity. Poisonings have followed both ingestion and topical application to abraded skin.

Phenol — This is carbolic acid. It is used in shaving creams and hand lotions. Obtained from coal tar, this material is a general disinfectant and anesthetic for the skin. Ingestion of even small amounts of this substance may cause nausea, vomiting, circulatory collapse, paralysis, convulsions and death, which results from respiratory failure. Fatal poisonings may also occur through skin absorption of phenol, although it is still widely used in commercial products. Swelling, pimples, hives and other more serious effects such as gangrene, burning and numbness have resulted from a topical application of just 1 percent phenol.

Sodium Hydroxide — This is a caustic soda that is used as an emulsifier in liquid facial cleansers, soaps, shampoos, cuticle removers, hair straighteners and creams. It is also used as a modifier for food starch, a glazing agent for pretzels and a peeling agent for tubers and skinned fruits. Because it is an alkali, it can cause dermatitis of the skin and scalp. Inhalation can cause lung damage.

Exercise — Essential to healthy skin is good blood circulation. A good way to achieve this maximum level of blood circulation is through a regular routine of exercise, but all too often, we forget about that one part of our skin that also could benefit from exercise: our face. Facial exercise can help to firm the muscles under the skin and stimulate the sebaceous glands into self-cleansing action, as well as supplying the face with a fresh supply of blood. Here are several exercises that stimulate and refresh the face:

• For the muscles around the eyes: With your head facing forward, look up at the ceiling and blink your eyelids rapidly, concentrating on bringing the lower lids up to meet the upper lids. Alternate this exercise with squeezing your eyelids tightly closed and then opening your eyes widely and moving your eyeballs in circles in both directions.

• For the cheeks: With your index finger resting on your nose, place the tip of your thumb in your mouth and then suck on it as hard as you can. Concentrate on moving your cheeks, not your mouth. This exercise will help to firm up the cheeks and contribute to that high-cheekboned look for which fashion models are envied.

• For the jaw and chin muscles: With the heel of your hand under your chin, try to open your mouth, while at the same time resisting the action by pushing upward with your hand. This exercise is useful in wiping out that unsightly double chin.

• For the muscles in the mouth: Open your mouth side, as if to scream, and then, with heavily exaggerated movements, mime the vowels "A, E, I, O, U, Y" several times. Concentrate on moving the muscles of your mouth. It's not necessary to do this aloud; just make sure you really exaggerate!

• For the neck and throat muscles: Lie on your bed with your head hanging face up over the side. Now, jut your jaw out and then open and close your mouth rapidly several times. You will be able to feel the muscles being pulled taut as you perform this exercise.

And of course, don't forget your regular exercise routine, either, or your well-balanced diet, with lots of fresh fruits and vegetables. Both are musts for healthy, radiant skin.

And, of course, a good diet, including something from each of the basic four food groups that we mentioned earlier, and regular exercise are also important factors in a good skin program. Let's look at the skin one more time.

There is very little absorbed into the skin from the outside. A little moisture perhaps, but virtually nothing in the way of nutrients, vitamins and minerals. Your skin relies on you to supply those elements, by way of a good diet. The healthier your diet, the more glowing your complexion should be. Likewise, a diet full of empty calories in the form of refined sugar often wreaks havoc with the skin, causing breakouts and a generally wan complexion.

Aren't facial exercises enough? No. In the section about exercise, we discussed the importance of blood circulation, so that those very important heart and lung muscles get worked properly. Well, good blood circulation is also important to the skin. Besides stimulating the sweat glands to empty out surface impurities, vigorous exercise allows the blood to remove the rest of those impurities from beneath the surface of the skin and supply it with fresh, nutrient-rich blood. You may notice that after a hard run or swim, your skin turns rosy. This is the blood's stimulating and cleansing action hard at work. Of course, your skin won't fall off if you don't exercise regularly, but if you are as concerned about your skin as you are about the rest of your body, you'll be twice as inclined to get out there and get moving every once in a while.

THE SEASONS OF YOUR SKIN

Depending on where you live, your skin will react differently to the changing weather conditions. Get to know your skin before you subject it to the ravages of winter wind and the harshness of summer sun. Many people fail to change their beauty routines with the seasons. Consult your skin to see if you should. Is it drying out too much when you sunbathe? Does your face get irritated and red after a long day of skiing in the cold? Plan your counterattack on weather's assaults wisely, because skin remembers: Everything harmful that happens to your skin will show up later.

The following is a list of helpful hints to assist your skin in surviving the summer sun. (Provided by Lia Schorr Skin Care, 527 Madison Ave., Suite 619, New York, NY 10022.)

- The sun is most intense between 11 a.m. and 3 p.m. If you must "bathe" in the rays, try to do so before 8 a.m. (yes, you can get a tan that early in the morning!) and after 3 p.m.

- Water and sand boost the burning potential of the sun.

- While clouds seem to mask the sun, they don't absorb the ultraviolet rays. Don't be fooled.

- Sun-block preparations usually have very little staying power. They wash off easily in water — or perspiration. Look for sunscreen preparations that contain PABA, zinc oxide or titanium oxide. Don't leave home without applying!

- No sun preparation will totally prevent the ultraviolet rays from hitting your skin. And remember to reapply often. A special stick-type sunscreen lip gloss is also a good bet.

- A non-greasy product is best. Oily preparations invite burning, itchy rashes and perspiration.

- Do not use perfume, antibacterial soap, medicated shampoos, antiseptic creams or highly perfumed hair conditioners. All can harm your skin while you're spending time in the sun.

- Dehydration is a by-product of too much sunning and warm-weather activity. Carry a spritzer filled with water — on the beach, on the tennis court or on the golf course.

- The summer-right accessories — Large sunglasses (green lenses are most protective), a large hat (to keep the sun — and your hair — off your face), all-cotton towels (absorbent and nonirritating), small pearl earrings (large metal ones hold heat) and poolside (or beachside) umbrella.

- The summer-savvy beauty routine — Switch to a light, water-based foundation. Those containing a sunscreen element are usually not as effective as we'd like to think. Apply a sunscreen preparation under your foundation. Don't use an alcohol-based astringent, it's too irritating. Instead, opt for a creamy cleanser and freshener. Your moisturizer should be richer, too.

- Sun reflectors are strictly taboo.

- Drink plenty of water when you're spending time in the sun. Alcohol and even fruit juice are too taxing on the system. Your body has to work too hard to digest the sugar.

- A good facial before you embark on a sun-filled escapade is recommended for its nourishing and deep-cleaning benefits. Plus, a good skin-care specialist can determine your skin type and can recommend a personalized course of action.

To cool a sunburn

- A cool bath (mix in three teaspoons of baking soda) for the body; cold tea bags over the eyes.

- A head-to-toe yogurt mask. Leave on for ten minutes then shower off with cool water.

- Drink a lot of water for hydration. Sweet drinks will only make you feel warmer.

- Baby powder helps reduce friction between your skin and clothes.

- Keep the body well moisturized to inhibit peeling.

- Don't rub your skin with a loofah or a towel.

For dry summer skin

- Apply mayonnaise to your face. Rinse off with cool water after ten minutes.

- Mash a banana (very ripe) with ½ teaspoon olive oil. Apply to your face, leave on for ten minutes, rinse. (You can substitute strawberries for the banana.)
- Take a milk bath (add three cups of whole milk to the tub).

For oily skin

- Plain yogurt mixed with wheat germ and honey makes a good mask. Leave on for ten minutes; rinse off with warm water.

For tired skin

- Apply compresses soaked in milk to tired eyes.
- Take a ginger bath. Grate a large ginger root and steep it in boiling water for twenty minutes. Strain the mixture. Add the liquid to a tubful of warm water. Place the grated ginger in a washcloth and "close" with a rubber band. Use this "spice sponge" to clean skin and stimulate circulation.
- Apply slices of pineapple or pear to your face. Leave on for ten minutes and then splash your face with cool water.

Winter can be brutal on your skin, but take heart — here are some ways to help your through. (Provided by Lia Schorr Skin Care, 527 Madison Ave., Suite 619, New York, N.Y. 10022.)

What are common winter beauty problems and what can be done about them?

Dry Skin. Cold air contains less moisture than warm air. Couple this with the fact that indoor heat is just as drying as outdoor cold, and what you have is winter skin; dry. Use a humidifier or a pan of water near your heating system to moisturize the air. Lowering your thermostat will help in the energy-conservation effort and the skin-conservation effort!

Chapped lips. Don't apply lipstick; it will dry them more. Don't pick and pull. Moisturize lips with your regular moisturizer several times a day, then apply lip gloss to protect. Better yet, use a lip balm with sunscreen (widely available in stick form).

Puffy red eyes. Soak six tea bags in boiling water. Apply three (lukewarm) to each closed eye. If your eyes are red from lack of sleep or too much reading, soak your face — eyes open — in a pot of distilled water for a minute.

What about washing with soap?

Soap is much too drying for even the oiliest skin; fatal for dry skin. "Soap dehydration" — the robbing of natural moisture from the skin — causes premature wrinkling. A mild, creamy cleanser is the better bet. Unlike soap, which collect bacteria, a bottled cleanser (to be applied with a cotton ball) is a germ-free way to cleanse.

Winter Masks, Potions and Notions

For starters, if you have to be out in the cold for a long period of time, wear a wool face mask — with cut-out spots for your eyes, nose and mouth — and clear your mind of all thoughts of vanity!

Face Masks (the other kind)
 1 cup plain yogurt (not low-fat, if possible)
 1 teaspoon fresh lemon juice
 1 teaspoon fresh orange juice
 1 teaspoon carrot juice

Mix, apply, leave on for ten minutes, splash with cool water.

Boil carrots and spinach in enough water to cover for about 1 hour. Puree, apply, relax, splash off with cool water.

For broken capillaries, mix chamomile powder (available from Lia Schorr) with buttermilk. Apply, leave on for 15 minutes, rinse off with warm water and cotton.

Raw potatoes or beets mashed with sour cream nourishes winter-dry skin.

Cleansing Lotions
 2 teaspoons honey
 1 teaspoon lemon juice
 4 teaspoons rose water
 5 teaspoons vodka

Mix together and let stand one week. Apply with cotton ball.

Use plain milk as a cleansing lotion when skin gets flaky. Apply with cotton ball — follow with a splash of distilled water or rose water.

Notions
Eat 3 carrots before going out into the cold. No matter how many layers of warm, wooly clothing you need to wear, always have your first layer (the one next to your skin) be 100 percent cotton.

Lia Schorr's "At Home" Facial
Step one: Cleansing
   Wash hands with soap and water.
   Apply liquid or creamy cleanser with a cotton ball, using up and down motions.
   Take another cotton ball, soaked in toning lotion, to finish cleansing and refresh skin.
Step two: Massage

   Take a thick cream in the palms of your hands, and with palms only massage your cheeks, in a circular motion, moving from center to hairline, then do your forehead.
   With index finger, pat cream gently around the eyes, moving from the corner of the eye to the nose. Never rub or pull.
   With index and middle fingers, massage nose and upper lips. Use all your fingers on your chin.
   For your neck, massage cream in with both hands, moving up and down.
   A massage stimulates circulation and tones muscles.
Step three: Steam and Moisture
   Place chamomile leaves in a pot of boiling water. Improvise a towel tent and steam your face to open pores. Follow with a nourishing mask. Remove after twenty minutes with lukewarm water. Finish with a light moisturizer.

YOUR LOVELY LOCKS: HAIR CARE

   Ah, what we would give for beautiful hair! Chances are, after you've finished gazing in the mirror at that gorgeous face of yours, the next feature you usually set your eyes on is your hair. And it's no wonder: Curly or straight, platinum blond or rosy brunette, long and streaming or short and pert, a woman's hair has long been a major sign of her overall beauty. We brush and comb it to death, curl it and unfurl it, run our hands through it (and let others run their hands through it), but sometimes, it just doesn't meet our expectations of beautiful hair.

   Be kind to your hair — it has a rough life. It's one of the only parts of our body that is almost always exposed to the elements, fragile though it is, and it takes lots of abuse, even from us. We wash it too much, fry it with blow dryers and curling irons, and let it get worn out by the sun and cold. And still we expect it to be bouncy, shimmery and thick. That's a tall order for one head of hair to fill. But with a little help from you, a little extra care, your hair can do wonderful things for your appearance.

   First, let's look at your hair's anatomy. Hair is much like skin, in that it is as complex in composition as the person who wears it. Your head contains approximately one hundred thousand to two hundred thousand hairs, each one growing and being nourished from its own follicle in the skin, your scalp. Each hair consists basically of two parts: the root and the shaft. The root is implanted in the scalp, while the shaft is the part that we actually see and touch. The root of

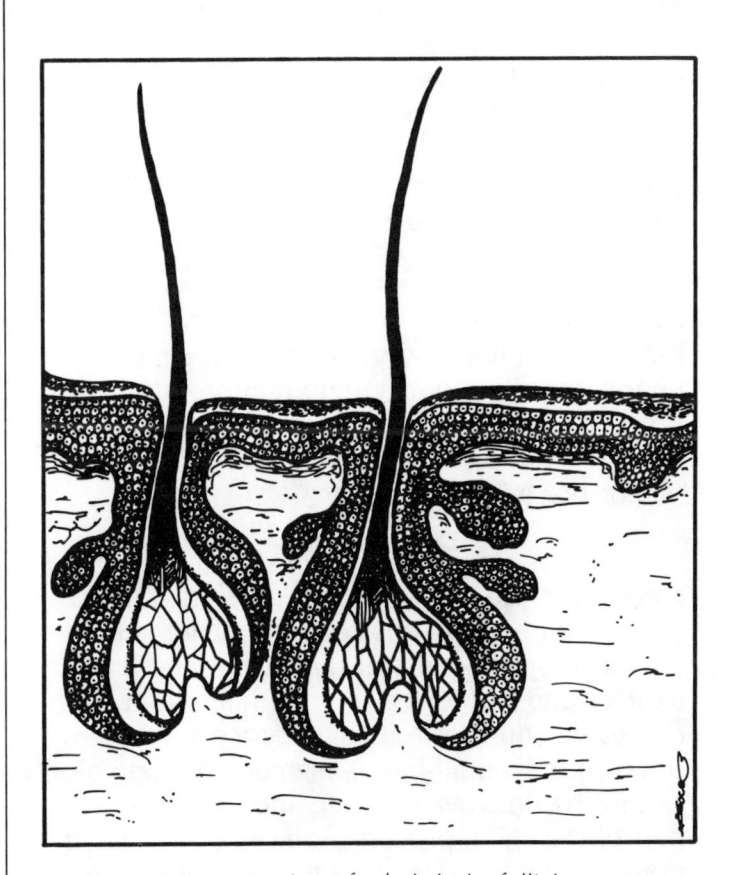

Microscopic cross-section of a hair in its follicle.

the hair ends in the hair bulb, an enlargement lodged in the hair follicle; in this bulb lies the papilla, which is richly supplied by blood vessels and nerve fibrils. It is in this region that the actual hair-growth process takes place.

All human hair goes through a cycle of death and replacement, but don't be alarmed: There are no nerve endings in hair with which to register pain, so it's a painless process. In fact, it's happening on your head at this very moment. When an individual hair cell dies, new cells begin to multiply in the papilla, the hair-growth region. As these new cells are formed, they begin to move toward the surface, pushing out the dead cells and replacing them with brand new hair. During this process, the new hair cells become elongated and toughened with a material called keratin; this is the part we see, the shaft.

The shaft consists of three main parts: the medulla (the inner core of the hair), the cortex (the main part of the hair shaft) and the cuticle (an outer layer of flat, overlapping scales). Normally, this cuticle is fairly smooth and light-reflective, making it shiny and soft. But abuse, overcare and things like permanents, color treatments and harsh shampoos can roughen and dull this outer layer, causing dryness and split ends (the "frizzies"). More about this later.

As in the skin, the scalp contains sebaceous glands, which secrete sebum. This natural lubricant normally flows along the hair shaft, imparting a natural luster to your hair. But certain conditions, like poor nutrition, improper care, hormonal imbalance, or disease, may interrupt normal sebum production, causing excessively oily or dry hair.

The color of your hair comes from pigmented granules in the cortex of the hair shaft. Determined by heredity, this coloring matter is produced by special cells at the base of the hair follicles and is injected into the hair when it becomes keratinized in its birth process. And once an individual hair is pigmented, that color cannot be destroyed. White and gray hair, as part of the aging process, appear when pigment does not get transferred to the cells of the cortex. In aging, this is a natural process largely determined by heredity.

The lifespan of the hairs on your head can range from months to several years, depending upon how healthy your hair and scalp are. When a woman gets older, often the follicles fail to produce normal hair cells, and consequently may cause thinning. But this process is a long time away, right? Not something we need to worry about just yet.

What we have just discussed are the ways in which hair is the same from person to person. But the wonderful thing about human hair is that, in many ways, it is so incredibly different on each of us. Long, lustrous and blond short, shiny and red, or sleek and chestnut brown, hair is one of the most individualizing characteristics of a woman — it is no wonder that it's the subject of such fancy as Goldilocks and Rapunzel. Hair can be one of the most beautifying aspects of your person, so be kind to it. Here are a few tips to help you keep your hair bouncy and beautiful:

• Once again, you can't stress diet enough. Yes, it even affects your hair, probably more than you think. Your hair and scalp, like every other part of your body, are made up of cells, which need to be properly nourished. And those cells rely on you to provide them with a diet that is high in vitamins and minerals. The basic building blocks are protein, carbohydrate and a touch of fat. A good diet will have marvelous effects on your hair.

• Make sure you are using quality products on your hair. More abuse is dealt to hair through dousing it with harsh shampoos and gummy creme rinses! Shop wisely for your hair-care products. Consult your hair stylist (if you have one); each person, according to her own hair type, will require a different hair-care program. But for starters, it is good to remember that hair likes protein-rich preparations, preferably ones that are pH balanced. (Your hair is slightly acid, and because shampoo is a detergent in a manner of speaking, it can often contain a lot of alkali, which is not so good for your hair.) Protein-rich shampoos and rinses can temporarily fill in the cracks and defects that can plague overly dry and damaged hair, making it smoother and thicker.

- Get a trim every now and then. This won't cause your hair to grow any faster, contrary to popular belief, but it will rid your locks of dry and split ends, and helps to keep it looking healthy and full.

- When combing your wet hair, use a wide-toothed comb, made of nylon or plastic. Using metal combs or brushing your hair with a bristled hair brush when it is wet may cause it to break and split.

- Don't scald your hair and scalp! Wash your hair in tepid to lukewarm water, but not in hot water. Besides burning yourself, this excessive heat can damage the hair shaft.

- When you wash your hair, you may think it's necessary to lather up two, even three times. Don't; you don't need squeaky-clean hair. If it squeaks, then chances are a lot of your hair's natural oils have been stripped away. You want to wash away the dirt and grime, not your hair's natural sheen. Too frequent shampooing can cause the same negative results: dull, dry, lifeless hair.

- If your hair is really dry, then maybe a conditioner will help. Protein conditioners (most especially those containing keratin) coat each strand of hair, making each thicker and stronger. In addition, conditioners will help to make your hair shiny by smoothing down the cuticle of each hair strand.

- Go ahead and style your hair pretty, but don't fry it to death with heat appliances. Blow dryers, curling irons and electric rollers (if you must use them) are real time-savers, but they can damage your hair if you're not careful. Here are a few things to remember if you are planning to work heat appliances into your beauty routine:

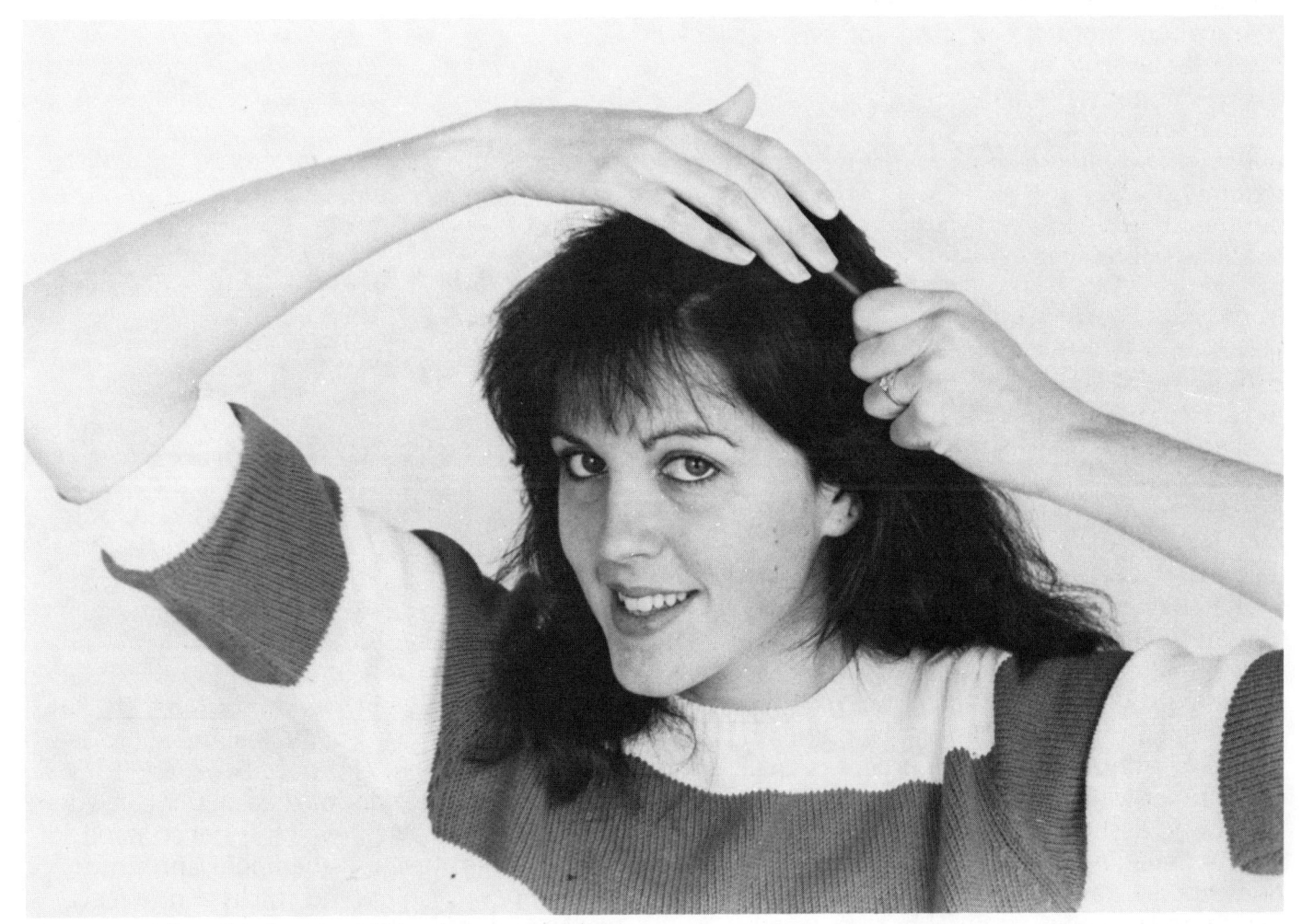

Try not to pull too hard on your hair when you comb it.

- Don't use your electric rollers every day. Give your hair a rest.

- Always use end papers with electric rollers. These dissipate some of that heat.

- Don't use your electric rollers when your hair is wet. You'll just fry those ends, and your style will not be as full and bouncy.

- If you use a curling iron, make sure your hair is completely dry before touching the iron to your hair. Take a blow dryer and move it freely about your hair until it is dry. The same goes for styling with your blow dryer and a brush. Let it dry; then style it with a brush.

- Constant pulling, brushing and combing can cause breaking and splitting — even cause your hair to fall out. That old "100 strokes" idea just doesn't pay; brush your hair enough to make it look nice, but don't overdo it. And if you wear your hair back in ponytails and buns, make sure that your style does not pull too much at the roots of your hair. Wear covered rubber bands so hair doesn't get pulled.

A "FITNESS" HAIR STYLE

Being that you are an active woman who exercises regularly, you will certainly want a hairstyle that will complement your fitness lifestyle.

Consequently, you probably won't have much use for expensive coiffures, which can be obtained only by visiting a stylist every week. And you probably won't be interested in a style that you must spend hours on every morning. You don't have that kind of time, and, anyway, it would fall to pieces as soon as you start running. You need a practical type of hairstyle, one that will move with you and cause as little hassle as possible.

Here are a few suggestions for hairstyles that work well with an active day:

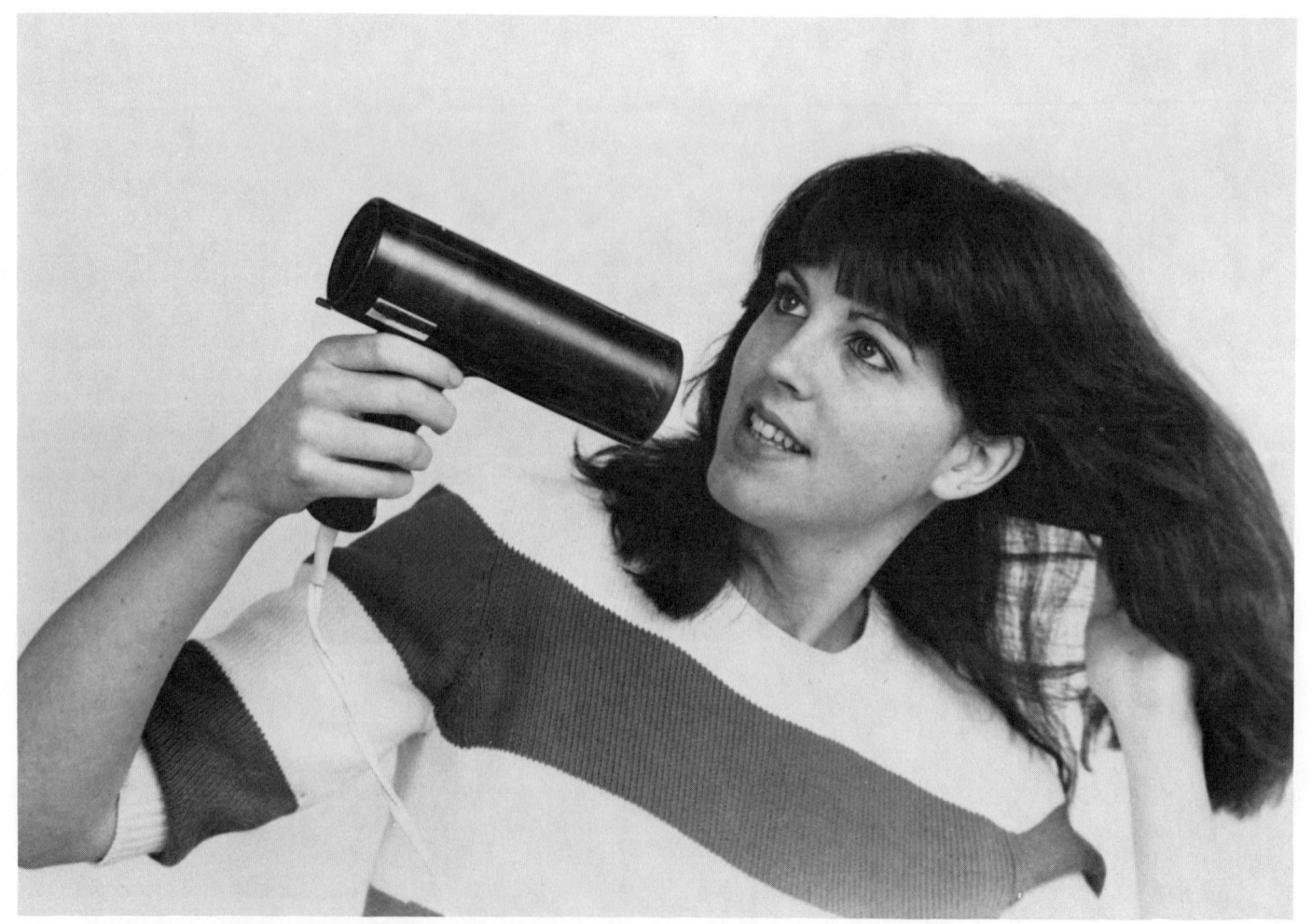

Blow dryers are convenient, but don't overuse them.

- Consider a natural body wave or permanent. Perms are easy to care for, and you won't have to mess with curling irons or blow dryers. If you do choose to have a perm, make sure your stylist is well-qualified. A poorly given perm may damage your hair, and will result in you having to spend even more money to have that damage corrected. The nice thing about having a natural body wave or perm is that you can go out for your run on your lunch hour, shower, and then let your hair dry naturally. The less you have to worry about your hair, the better.

- If you can't bring yourself to part with your lovely long locks, spice them up with ribbons and bows. Long hair handles exercise much better if it is tied back and out of your way. Tie it back in a long ponytail with a ribbon (use covered rubber bands, so that you don't cause splitting and breakage), or put it in a knot at the top of your head. Depending on how much time you want to spend working with your hair, you may or may not want a style that involves a lot of curling.

- Long hair can also be covered and kept out of your face with a bandanna. Not only are bandannas stylish right now, but they help your hair by keeping the sun off it; hair tends to dry out and break when it is exposed for too long to hot, harsh sunlight.

- Short cuts can be very flattering also, and they fit perfectly into a fitness lifestyle. They don't need much care — perhaps a little touching up with the blow dryer — and they are comfortable, especially when you get hot and sweaty during a workout or after a long day in the sun.

PICTURE-PERFECT POSTURE

Remember how Mom always used to yell at you when you slouched in your chair? "Stand up straight!" she would command; "You'll get curvature of the spine."

Well, she may not have been right about curvature of the spine, but she was right about realizing the importance of good posture. Good posture is a key to a really nice figure — it's essential, in fact. Even the fittest of bodies will look listless and out of shape if it is not carried properly. Think of someone you know who has very bad posture. Do you consider that person attractive? Fit? Probably not.

Don't spoil the wonderful effects of exercise on your body by exhibiting poor posture. An erect carriage not only looks good but allows for better blood circulation, prevents fatigue and stress on the joints and the spine, and implies to strong will and self-confidence on your part. Be conscious of your posture; it's an important element of your appearance that should not go unnoticed. Here are a few hints for keeping your posture as lovely as possible:

- A lot of our posture problems are created by the way we sit. Pretend you are watching yourself from a hidden camera. How are you sitting? Up nice and straight, or slouching? When you are sitting, make every effort to keep your entire back against the back of the chair. Don't sit with your rear on the front of the chair and your neck resting on the back. Keep the crown of your head parallel with the ceiling — nice and tall, like a queen on a throne. Don't cross your legs while you are sitting, either. Sometimes crossing your legs tends to make you slouch down in your chair.

- When you stand, you should be able to draw an imaginary line from your ear to just in front of your ankle bone. It's a good idea not to stand for too long of a period, and especially, avoid ill-fitting shoes — fashionable or not.

- A good posture exercise is the Invisible Chair. Stand against a wall, with your back straight. Now, slowly, lower your body and adjust your legs so that you are "sitting" with your knees bent out in front of you and your back straight against the wall. Hold this position for thirty seconds.

- When you are walking, look straight ahead, keeping the crown of your head parallel with the ceiling. Don't look down at your feet or the ground unless you really have to; this tends to make you walk with your shoulders hunched over, and can lead to bad posture. Keep your shoulders back, and be aware of what your body looks like while you are walking.

FIGURE MAINTENANCE

Posture — Sitting

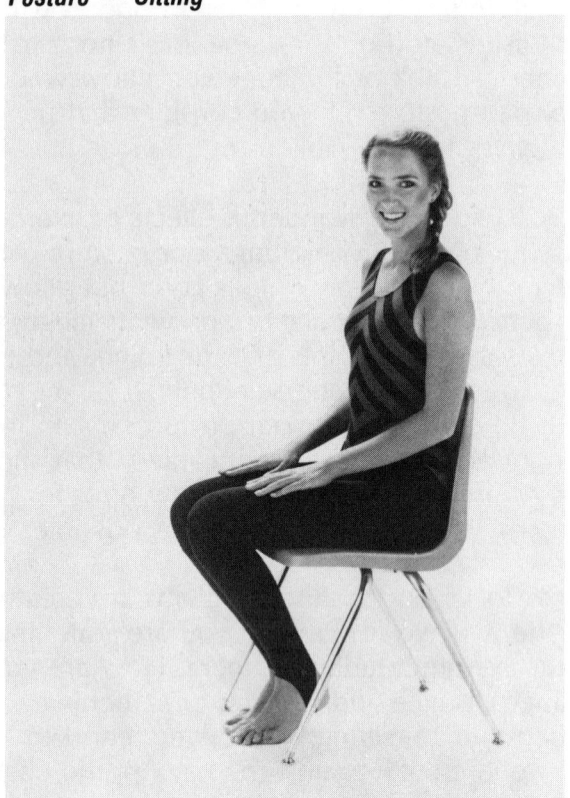

a. Correct posture while sitting.

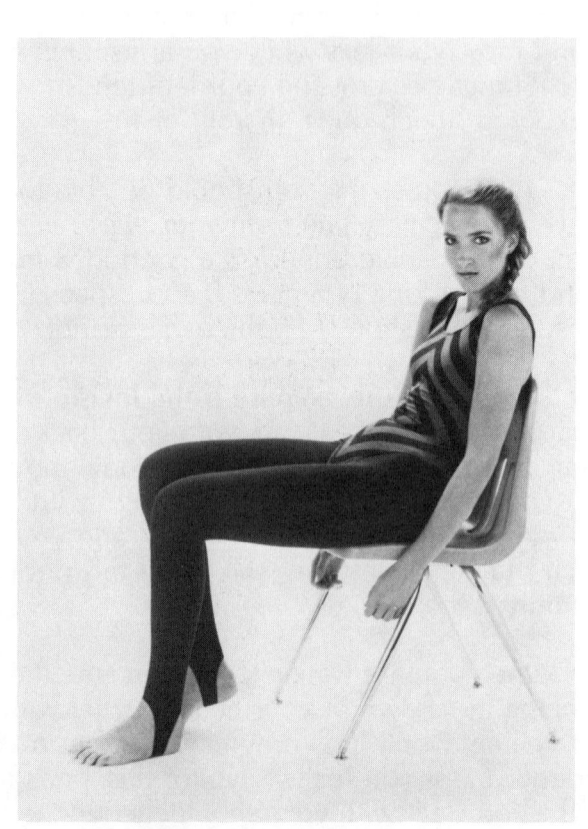

b. Incorrect posture while sitting.

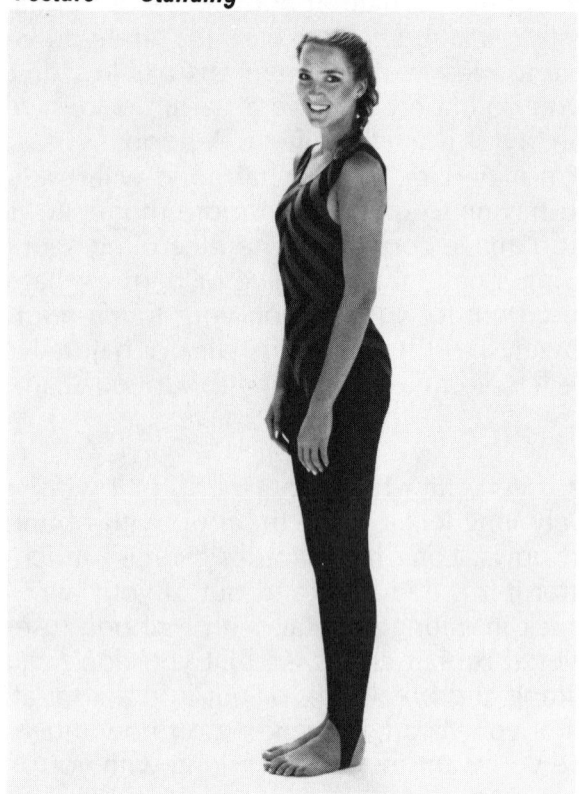

Posture — Standing

a. Correct posture while standing.

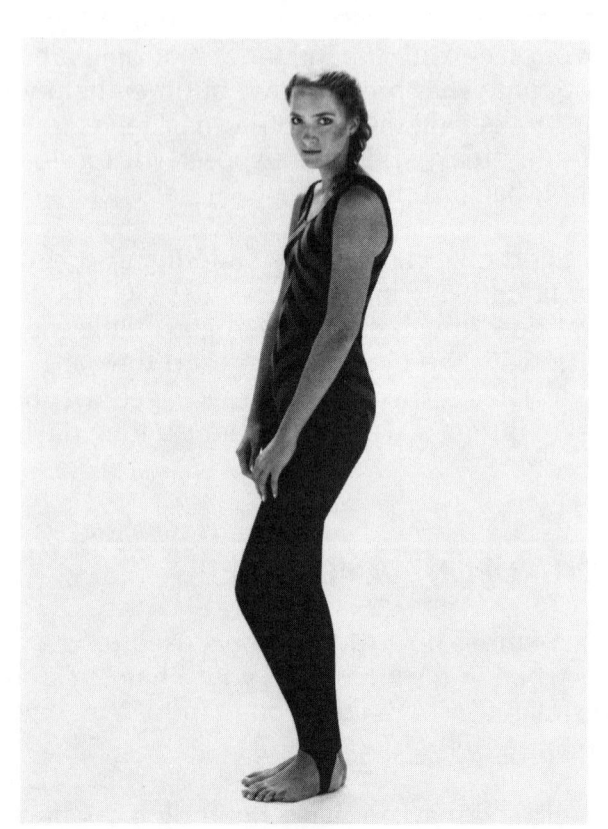

b. Incorrect posture while standing.

Appearance 81

Posture — Lifting

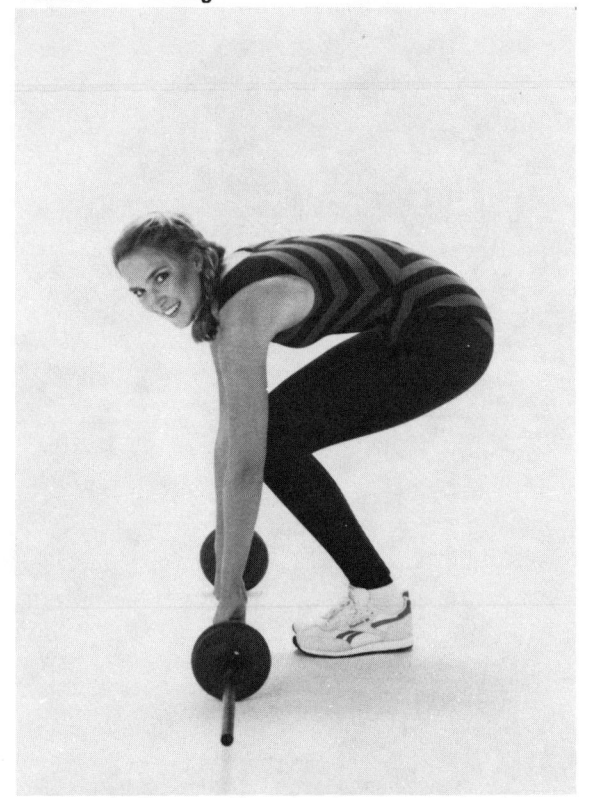

a. Bend at the knees when you lift a heavy object. Use your legs, not your back.

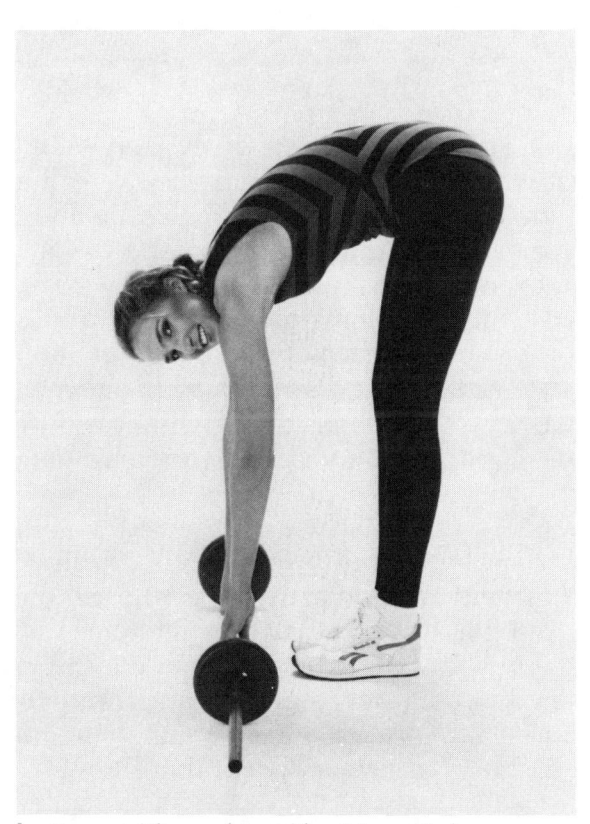

b. Do not lift an object like this, with legs straight. It puts excessive stress on the back.

Posture — Sleep

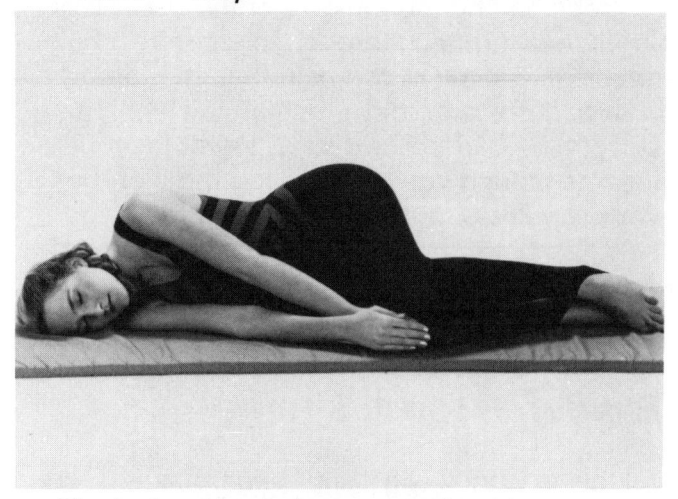

The fetal position is the most comfortable position for most people during sleep.

INVISIBLE CHAIR

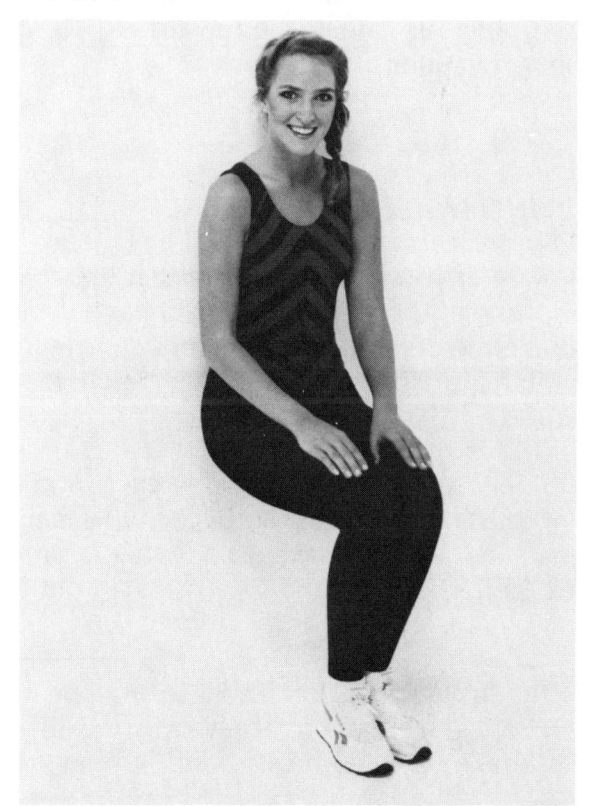

A good way to improve back posture is to pretend you are sitting in a chair against a wall.

Strengthening the muscles of the back, legs, shoulders and neck through exercise will help to alleviate some of the pain that goes along with bad posture, and eventually will help to correct the bad posture itself. Don't let yourself look as though you are carrying the world on your shoulders. Straighten up, and realize the benefits, both physical and mental, that good posture can have.

BEING FIT IS LOOKING FIT

How you look is a major determinant of your overall health and fitness. Getting back to that old car, what's the use of having a great running engine, a tip-top-shape transmission and a fantastic set of tires if you've got a paint job that looks like something your kid brother might have done in nursery school? Or if the inside looks as though a tornado just passed through? Show off the wonderful benefits of your fit figure by accentuating your outer beauty. Wear clothes that flatter your figure, and take care of your skin and hair. Don't hide your fitness — put it on display for all the world to see. After all, one of the rewards of being fit is being beautiful!

PUTTING IT ALL TOGETHER

Now — if you haven't written that letter yet, go do it, right now. That is, if you have decided to make the commitment to keep your figure youthful and vibrant through living a life of fitness.

No one said it was going to be easy. But, then, isn't it worth it? Isn't it worth it to feel energetic and alive, to have a body that is strong, sleek (and sexy, too), and to possess an outlook on life that is positive and carefree?

In the first segment of this Fit Instructional Book Series, we have basically overviewed what it takes to keep healthy and fit: good diet;

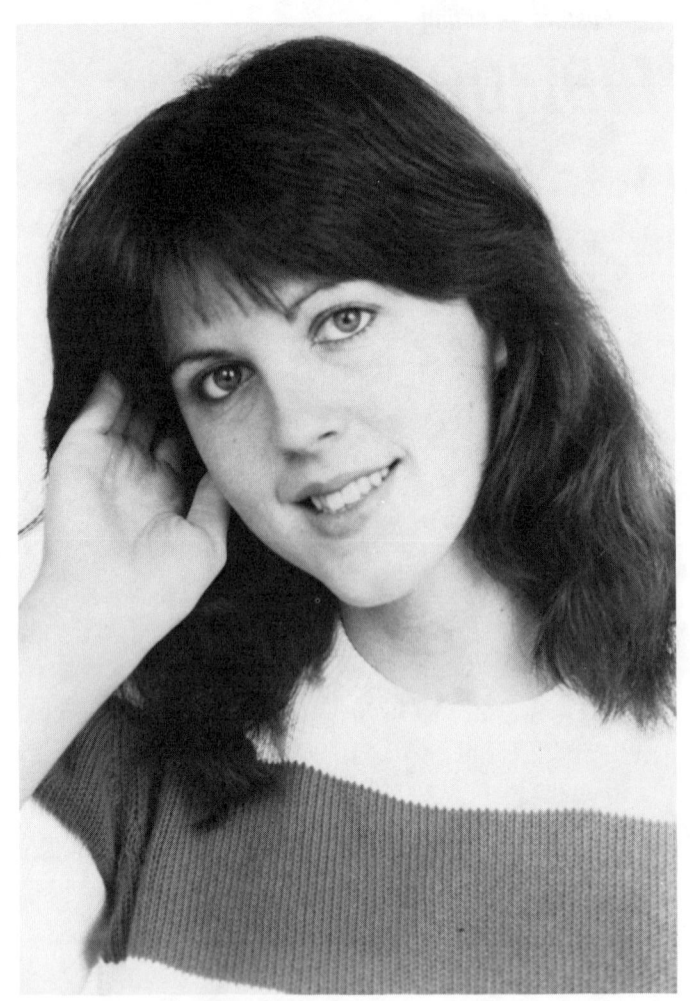

The finished product.

regular, vigorous exercise; an awareness of what is going on inside our bodies as well as outside; and a positive mental attitude and peace of mind. And you really can't feel all the benefits of any of these basic fitness requirements without helping them to work in unison — one is just as important to a fit figure and lifestyle as the next. Put them all together and — wow! — you'll knock yourself out with the results (and you'll knock everyone else out, too!).

So, go ahead! Jot down that letter in the boldest and firmest handwriting you can muster. And make it a lifelong commitment. Each year, on your birthday, copy that letter all over again. As you grow older, let your commitment mature with you. Make a beautiful figure, and a life of fitness, a neverending proposition!

BIBLIOGRAPHY

Bailey, Covert, *Fit or Fat?*. Boston: Houghton Mifflin, Co., 1978.

Berkeley Food Co-op, *Health Food Book*. Mountain View, Calif.: Anderson World Inc., 1982.

Couch, Jean with Weaver, Nell, *Runner's World Yoga Book*. Mountain View, Calif.: Runner's World Books, 1979.

Francko, David, *Health Club Book*. Mountain View, Calif.: Anderson World Inc., 1980.

Frank, Diana, *Runner's World No Time To Cook Cookbook*. Mountain View, Calif.: Runner's World Books, 1981.

Hastings, Fadiman, Gordon, *Health for the Whole Person*. Boulder, Colo.: Westview Press, 1980.

Jackson, Douglas, M.D., and Pescar, Susan, *The Young Athlete's Health Handbook*. Ontario: Beaverbooks, Don Mills, 1981.

Johnson, Timothy, M.D., and Goldfinger, Stephen, M.D., *The Harvard Medical School Health Letter Book*. New York: Warner Books (a division of Warner Communications), 1981.

Kaye, Frederick S., *A Dietary Guideline*. Published in coordination with the Family Practice Program of Tallahassee, Fla., Regional Medical Center, 1981.

Lawrence, Ned, Rajala, John and Sciutto, Carole, *Total Fitness for the Working Person*. Dublin, Calif.: Corporate Fitness Inc., 1980.

Sheehan, George, M.D., *The Encyclopedia of Athletic Medicine*. Mountain View, Calif.: *Runner's World* magazine, World Publications, 1972.

Stallings, James O., M.D., *Beauty Is My Business*. New York: Frederick Fell Publishers Inc., 1982.

Ullyot, Joan, M.D., *Women's Running*. Mountain View, Calif.: World Publications, 1976.

U.S. Dietary Guidelines, Nutrition and Your Health. Washington, D.C.: United States Department of Agriculture, Bulletin No. 232.

Weaver, Nell, *Runner's World Stretching Book*. Mountain View, Calif.: Anderson World Inc., 1981.

Yeager, Trisha, *The California Beauty Book*. San Francisco: Harbor Publishing Co., 1981.

CREDITS

MODELS

Sandra Rothbucher appears in Chapter 2 and Chapter 5 exercise routines.

Andrea Shyne appears on pages 68 (left), 70, 78 and 82.

Michele Kelly appears in Chapter 2 (walking, bicycling, roller skating, jumping rope).

Joan Goggin appears on page 68 (right).

PHOTOGRAPHERS

Exercise routines and the four basic food group photos are by *Runner's World* staff photographer David Keith.

Skip Heine photo, page 61.

Julian Baum photo, page 48.

THE *FIT SELF-IMPROVEMENT SERIES* IS PUBLISHED BY THE EDITORS OF *FIT* MAGAZINE. TO RECEIVE *FIT* EVERY MONTH, SEND $ 14.95 TO:
FIT MAGAZINE
1400 STIERLIN ROAD
MOUNTAIN VIEW, CA
94043